Research at the Durham
Veterans Affairs Medical Center
(1953–2005)

Research at the Durham
Veterans Affairs Medical Center
(1953–2005)
An Overview

Joseph C. Greenfield, Jr., M.D.

From the Department of Medicine,
Division of Cardiology, Duke University
and Durham Veterans Affairs Medical Centers,
Durham, N.C.

Supported in part by the Institute for Medical
Research, Durham Veterans Affairs Medical Center
and The Greenfield Scholars Endowment,
Duke University.

To Dave

Best Wishes

JfG 2009

Joe Gfd

CAROLINA ACADEMIC PRESS
Durham, North Carolina

LCCN: 2009927595
ISBN: 978-1-59460-746-2

Carolina Academic Press
700 Kent Street
Durham, NC 27701
Telephone (919) 489-7486
Fax (919) 493-5668
www.cap-press.com

Printed in the United States of America

Dedication

Although a number of individuals have made major contributions to the Research Program at the DVA, Burley Houston McCraw clearly stands out as the primary guiding force. As the Administrative Officer for Research and Development, Burley steered the fledgling program during its major developmental phase. Without his untiring effort, undoubtedly the program could not have achieved the current level of success.

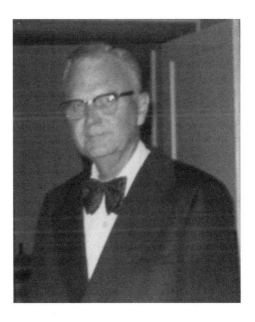

Contents

Preface   ix

Acknowledgments   xi

Beginning   3

Investigators   5

Anesthesiology   7

Basic Sciences   9

Dentistry   13

Medicine/Cardiology   15

Medicine/Dermatology   19

Medicine/Endocrinology   21

Medicine/Gastroenterology   23

Medicine/General Medicine   27

Medicine/Geriatrics   31

Medicine/Hematology and Medical Oncology   35

Medicine/Infectious Diseases   37

Medicine/Nephrology   39

Medicine/Neurology   41

Medicine/Pulmonary   43

Medicine/Rheumatology and Immunology   47

Mental Health   49

Ophthalmology   53

Pathology and Laboratory Medicine   55

Radiology   57

Surgery/General Surgery   59

Surgery/Cardiothoracic Surgery   61

Surgery/Neurosurgery   63

Surgery/Orthopaedics   65

Surgery/Urology   67

Summation   69

Centers   75
     HSR&D   75
     GRECC   84
Facilities   87
Funding   93
Administration   97
Future   99
Sources   101

Preface

This overview of the research carried out at the Durham Veterans Affairs Hospital (DVA)* from its inception through 2005 had a somewhat unusual—bizarre—genesis. Marguerite T. Hays, M.D. was commissioned by the Central Office Research Service to write a comprehensive two-volume history of research endeavors of the Veterans Administration. The plan was to have one volume contain an overview of research from a number of individual medical centers, including the DVA. I was asked by the Associate Chief of Staff (ACOS) for Research and Development, J. Brice Weinberg, M.D. to prepare a response. For reasons not entirely clear, I agreed. A manuscript was completed and submitted to Dr. Hays in 2003. Without explanation, approximately one year later, the project was cancelled abruptly. This situation was discussed with John D. Shelburne, M.D., Ph.D., Chief of Staff, and Dr. Weinberg. Since the initial manuscript contained important historical information, a proposal was developed to significantly expand its scope and to publish a revised overview. After they both volunteered to be very supportive of this venture, I "elected" to proceed.

The original manuscript gave a brief synopsis of the research efforts of a few selected investigators as examples of the research program, but was, by no means, exhaustive. In deciding on the format for this expanded overview, an effort was made to catalogue all of the investigators who carried out independent funded research for a significant period of time at the DVA and to document their subsequent careers. These data illustrate the fact that these individuals made major contributions both to research and to

---

* DVA will be used throughout the text to designate the facility currently known as the Durham Veterans Affairs Medical Center.

Duke Medical Center (DUMC) as well as to a number of other academic institutions.

In preparing this manuscript, most of the historical information was obtained through personal communication with a number of individuals[1]. Unfortunately, the majority of the historical records are no longer available locally, having been transferred to Central Office where, if they exist, are in an unavailable format. Thus, the only recourse was to depend on hearsay. Obviously, relying on the potentially faulty memory of colleagues and myself is by no means a perfect way to retrieve comprehensive data. Undoubtedly, investigators who should have been included were not. For these inadvertent errors, I apologize. However, the presented material does codify a wealth of information which otherwise would have been lost.

Acknowledgments

The good-natured effort of Bettie C. Houston, who typed the multiple drafts of this manuscript, is gratefully appreciated.

Judith C. Rembert was responsible for amassing, collating, and cataloging the data, as well as providing invaluable editorial assistance.

The staff of Medical Media, Durham Veterans Affairs Medical Center, was responsible for the illustrations.

Research at the Durham
Veterans Affairs Medical Center
(1953–2005)

Beginning

By the time the newly opened DVA was dedicated, April 19, 1953, its future as an outstanding research facility had been firmly established.[2] The primary reason responsible for this success is summarized in the report of a site visit carried out on May 15, 1968 to evaluate the overall research program.[3]

"Research scientists and clinical investigators at the Durham VA Hospital appear to have been selected by a rather unique process, in that each appointment of the staff physician at the VA Hospital was made only after whole hearted endorsement by related departments at Duke University. This has resulted in extremely close ties of all professional personnel with Duke University and we found no VA scientist or physician who did not have an appointment to a University department.

This arrangement has resulted in a very high standard of competence of the VA professional personnel which in turn has assured an extremely effective research program."[3]

Recognizing the opportunity for fostering research at this new facility, several of the Department Chairmen at DUMC recruited research scientists as key members of the initial administrative staff of the DVA. They, in turn, set about including research as an integral component of the hospital mission. In selecting investigators, performing the highest quality research was of paramount importance; however, an additional factor was the requirement that the individual assure excellence in patient care. In fact, from the inception, the research program provided a rich milieu whereby these outstanding physician scientists impacted positively on the care of the Veteran patients.

Investigators

As with any human endeavor, ultimate success depends entirely on the quality of the people involved. Over the past five decades, the DVA Research Program has been blessed by having a number of outstanding scientists directing the research laboratories. Clearly, not only are the principal scientists important, but the quality of the laboratory technicians and other ancillary personnel are key factors in the ultimate outcome. As a group, these individuals were, and are, outstanding. They performed a major role in fulfilling the research mission.

A major function of every research laboratory is to foster the development of young scientists. The overwhelming majority of the investigators at the DVA performed admirably in this task. A complete listing of the students, doctoral candidates and physicians who received research training at the DVA has not been attempted. However, the aggregate numbers have been extraordinary. In fact, many of the investigators described in this text received their initial research training at this facility.

Although it is beyond the scope of this presentation to detail the research at the DVA in its entirety, the key investigators are described.[4–6] In order to be included, an investigator either had independent involvement in research for several years or directed at least one clinical trial or cooperative study. In addition, each individual received significant research funding through either the VA system or from extramural sources. These investigators are grouped by their specialty (and when appropriate, subspecialty) and presented in semi-chronological order. For those who either served or are currently in an administrative academic position, their highest rank is listed. Individuals who currently are involved in research at the DVA are identified by an asterisk after their name. The material usually includes a very short general overview of their research carried out primarily at the DVA; however, comprehensive details and bibliographic citations are not given. When applicable, the contributions of these individuals and their research to the DVA patient care mission are highlighted.

At the end of each group, the percent pursuing a predominantly academic career either at DUMC or elsewhere is provided. In addition, there is an estimate of the total number of scientific publications authored, or co-authored, by these investigators during their entire career. Since a number of manuscripts have been authored, as well as co-authored, by several of the investigators, the aggregate number may be erroneously high.

There are a large number of physicians whose primary function at the DVA was the clinical care of the Veteran patients. As a group, they formed the backbone of the Clinical Services. Many of these individuals have participated in clinical research and made important contributions to the research enterprise, including publishing research manuscripts. By adhering to the criteria which defined a research investigator, the names of these individuals cannot be listed. However, a great debt of gratitude is owed to them for their contributions to the research program at the DVA.

Anesthesiology

During the first three decades, the Anesthesiology Service functioned through the Department of Surgery and did not have physicians primarily at the DVA. Robert N. Sladen, M.D. became Chief of the Anesthesiology Service in the 1980s. An extraordinary clinical teacher and critical care physician, Dr. Sladen conducted numerous clinical trials focused on perioperative organ dysfunction and monitoring, focusing on kidney damage, blood pressure management, and temperature changes associated with cardiac surgery. Dr. Sladen can be credited with making research activities a vital part of the DVA Anesthesiology Service mission. In 1992, Jonathan B. Mark, M.D.* succeeded Dr. Sladen as Service Chief and further supported and developed a vibrant anesthesiology research program. One of the earliest investigators and collaborators with Dr. Sladen was Joel S. Goldberg, M.D.*, who performed some of the initial clinical trials at the DVA in the 1980s.

Dr. Mark has investigated perioperative hemodynamic monitoring techniques, including noninvasive cardiac output monitoring and transesophageal echocardiography. In addition, he is evaluating the safety of moderate sedation practice and designing improved training of clinical providers through point of care high fidelity medical simulation. This work is supported by the VA National Center for Patient Safety, which has funded Dr. Mark and colleagues to establish a VA Patient Safety Center of Inquiry in Durham. Rebecca A. Schroeder, M.D.* and Atilio Barbeito, M.D.* are co-investigators in this project, and they have also pursued other clinical trials while at the DVA, focusing on perioperative embolic events and other adverse perioperative outcomes.

Terri G. Monk, M.D.* has investigated the etiology and mechanism underlying perioperative cognitive dysfunction. Currently, studies are being carried out to define the intraoperative determinants of perioperative morbidity through analysis of electronic anesthesia records.

Shahar Bar-Yosef, M.D.* is investigating the outcome of occult adrenal insufficiency in critically ill patients and the role of perioperative temperature management in preventing cognitive dysfunction following heart surgery.

In the 1990s and early 2000s, a number of other clinical investigators held competitive grant funding for clinical trials at the DVA. Thomas F. Slaughter, M.D. studied the mechanisms for perioperative coagulopathy in patients undergoing cardiac surgery. His colleague working in the field of perioperative hemostasis, Gautam M. Sreeram, M.D., explored the role of a point of care platelet function analyzer and desmopressin therapy in identifying patients at risk for perioperative hemorrhage following heart surgery. Ellen M. Flanagan, M.D. evaluated the outcome of surgical procedures in elderly patients who have concomitant DNR orders.

Two other outstanding investigators were part of the Anesthesiology Service in the past decade. Laura E. Niklason, M.D., Ph.D. is known internationally for her pioneering work involving tissue engineering of artificial blood vessels, and Mihai V. Podgoreanu, M.D.* is a leading investigator in the field of perioperative genomics and predictors of adverse events.

All of these 12 investigators have pursued academic careers with eight remaining at DUMC. Approximately 366 manuscripts have been authored or co-authored by these individuals.

Basic Sciences

An example of the appointment of an outstanding scientist which led to the development of a long-term research program as well as significantly impacting on the Clinical Services, was made by Philip Handler, Ph.D. (Chairman, Department of Biochemistry, DUMC). The DVA Clinical Services required expertise in the use of radioisotopes—primarily radioactive iodine for the diagnosis and treatment of thyroid disease. Dr. Handler obtained an appointment for Henry Kamin, Ph.D., a graduate student in his laboratory who was studying microsomal cytochromes, to be responsible for this function. Several scientists, both M.D. and Ph.D., participated in this endeavor and the Nuclear Medicine Service came into existence. James O. Wynn, M.D. provided critical input in the initial phase of this effort. Later, Ralph J. Gorton, M.D. expanded the capabilities of this Service and, in addition, carried out research in both thyroid and cardiac imaging.

Dr. Kamin developed his own basic science research program and recruited Ronald C. Greene, Ph.D. This group was initially housed in the only dedicated research space available when the DVA facility opened: Building 10 (Figure 1), a 2500 sq. ft. building which contained reasonably adequate wet laboratory facilities. Dr. Greene maintained an independent and well-funded basic biochemical research laboratory at the DVA for nearly 40 years. Dr. Greene, Harvey J. Sage, Ph.D. and Lewis M. Siegel, Ph.D. (Vice Provost and Dean of the Graduate School, DUMC) became known as the basic sciences group of investigators. They not only carried out excellent basic research in a variety of different areas involving cellular metabolism and function, but were responsible for mentoring a number of Ph.D. candidates as well as providing invaluable advice and methodological expertise to many of the physician scientists.

More recently, an independent basic science investigator, R. Neal Shepherd, Ph.D.*, studied contraction characteristics in isolated cardiac myocytes.

One of the most important, but unexpected, contributions resulting from the Nuclear Medicine Program was the appointment of Burley H. McCraw as the Radiation Safety Officer. Burley's initial efforts were directed primarily toward the safe use of radioisotopes. However, his penchant for research administration soon became quite obvious. In short order, he became responsible for administrating the basic sciences group. His success in this endeavor led to Burley's appointment as the Administrative Officer for Research and Development for the entire DVA research program. In this role, he was clearly one of the major factors in promoting the outstanding growth. He continued in this position, fostering the development of the research program until the time of his retirement in 1982.

All of these six investigators have had long-term academic careers with five remaining at DUMC. Approximately 244 publications were authored or co-authored by these individuals.

Figure 1

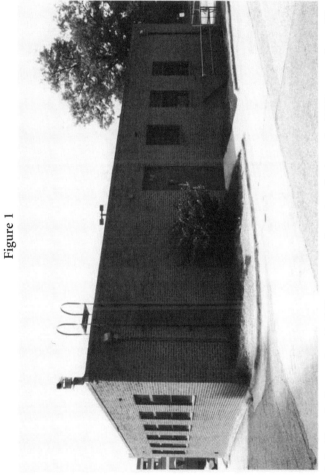

This research facility, designated as Building 10, was functional when the DVA opened—still going strong.

Dentistry

Alan F. Shernoff, D.D.S.* was the principal investigator of a Co-operative study evaluating dental implants in a diabetic population. The data indicated a similar success rate for diabetic vs. non diabetic patients.

Medicine/Cardiology

Prior to the opening of the DVA, Eugene A. Stead, Jr., M.D. (Chairman, Department of Medicine, DUMC) appointed James V. Warren, M.D., a widely recognized cardiovascular physiologist and cardiologist, to head the Medicine Service. In turn, Dr. Warren recruited a number of young cardiovascular physician scientists: Harold T. Dodge, M.D., Arnold M. Weissler, M.D. (Chairman, Department of Medicine, Wayne State Medical Center) and E. Harvey Estes, Jr., M.D. (Chairman, Department of Family Medicine, DUMC). They immediately initiated active programs in cardiovascular research.

Dr. Dodge's area of interest was the study of ventricular function in man using angiographic measurement of ventricular volumes. Dr. Weissler investigated the multiple factors which influence vasomotion in man and defined several of the mechanisms of syncope. Dr. Estes' primary research interest was in electrocardiography using the vector approach. In addition, he was responsible for acquiring the Cooperative Lipid Lab for the DVA. This laboratory carried out major research and clinical functions for both the local and national VA program for a number of years.

Joseph C. Greenfield, Jr., M.D.* (Chairman, Department of Medicine, DUMC) led a cardiovascular research laboratory for three and one-half decades. Initially, this research was performed in the Cardiac Catheterization Laboratory measuring instantaneous blood pressure-flow relationships in the human ascending aorta. This research attracted a number of outstanding young investigators who essentially ran the Cardiac Catheterization Laboratory for greater than 25 years. Drs. Jerome Ruskin and Abe Walston, II carried out a number of clinical studies primarily involving patients on the Cardiac Care Unit.

In addition, detailed studies of factors which regulate coronary blood flow were carried out in an awake canine model which simulated the human cardiovascular system in both health and disease states. A number of physician trainees participated in these studies and two became outstanding independent and long-term VA investigators: Frederick R. Cobb, M.D.* and Robert J. Bache, M.D. Two of the seven Ph.D. candidates who finished their graduate work in the laboratory, Judith C. Rembert, Ph.D.* and Philip A. McHale, Ph.D. continued research for a number of years.

Dr. Cobb's research at the DVA involved the study of canine myocardial blood flow during a variety of ischemic situations. This work led to the development of a unique model to define the relationship between myocardial ischemia and myocardial infarction. In addition, Dr. Cobb carried out extensive studies of the factors involved in vasomotion of the major coronary vessels. This investigation led to the development of strategies to define the presence and progression of atherosclerotic vascular disease. Also, he studied the efficacy of various modalities employed in the therapy of congestive heart failure in patients.

Dr. Bache transferred his activities to the Minneapolis VA Hospital where he continues his very productive investigative career in cardiac pathophysiology.

Patrick A. McKee, M.D. (Chairman, Department of Medicine, University of Oklahoma Health Sciences Center) studied the basic mechanisms involved in clotting with a particular emphasis on factors which control the conversion of fibrinogen to fibrin.

Robert P. Bauman, M.D. functioned both as a basic investigator studying myocardial blood flow and directed a clinical trial evaluating atherectomy.

A. Alan Chu, M.D. studied the distribution of thallium-201 in normal, ischemic and infarcted myocardium.

Mitchell W. Krucoff, M.D.* developed and tested a number of novel monitoring systems to enhance the diagnosis of cardiac ischemic syndromes. More than a thousand patients have been involved in two dozen clinical trials in evaluating this technology. Intangible human tools and capacities such as relaxation, music, imagery, touch and prayer have undergone the scientific study of the use of these modalities in peri-procedural patient management.

Using primarily a porcine model, Richard S. Stack, M.D. studied the pathophysiology of the response in the coronary vasculature to injury produced by angioplasty and the placement of intravascular stents. He developed a perfusion balloon catheter which significantly reduced the complications of angioplasty.

Intervention/revascularization strategies have been examined by Kenneth G. Morris, M.D.* in both VA Cooperative and industry sponsored studies.

Andrea Natale, M.D. performed a number of clinical studies to define the role of invasive electrophysiology in the management of patients with atrial and ventricular arrhythmias.

Brian H. Annex, M.D.* has carried out a number of basic studies to define the vascular cellular function in response to growth factors. In addition, he has developed a research program to evaluate and treat DVA patients with peripheral vascular disease.

Recently, Mark P. Donahue, M.D.* has initiated in-depth studies to quantitate genetic abnormalities in patients with myocardial disease.

Of these 17 investigators, 12 have continued a long-term academic career with seven remaining at DUMC. One individual is in industry. Approximately 1563 publications have been authored or co-authored by these individuals.

Medicine/Dermatology

Although the physicians in Dermatology provided excellent clinical care and carried out clinical research during the initial two decades, basic investigation of the immunology of dermatologic diseases awaited the programmatic input of Drs. Jegasothy and Hall.

Brian V. Jegasothy, M.D. (Chairman, Department of Dermatology, University of Pittsburgh) focused on the immunology of T cells. Dr. Jegasothy's laboratory was instrumental in characterizing T cell factors that inhibited lymphocyte responses. Dr. Jegasothy also made important contributions to our understanding of cutaneous T cell lymphoma. These included characterizing the malignant T cells, and contributing to the discovery of the role of retroviruses in some forms of T cell malignancy.

Russell P. Hall, III, M.D.* (Chief, Dermatology, DUMC) carried out research focused on understanding the pathogenesis of immunologically mediated blistering diseases including dermatitis herpetiformis (DH), bullous pemphigoid and pemphigus vulgaris. His work has helped to characterize the relationship between the mucosal immune response in the gut and the development of the skin lesions of DH and contributed to the understanding of the antibody-antigen interactions that occur in patients with pemphigoid and pemphigus.

Both of these investigators have had long-term academic careers (one remaining at DUMC) and authored or co-authored approximately 146 manuscripts.

Medicine/Endocrinology

The initial primary role of the endocrinologists was the diagnosis and treatment of thyroid dysfunction. As such, these physicians were involved in the use of radioisotopes to evaluate and treat thyroid abnormalities. James O. Wynn, M.D. studied a number of factors which controlled the level of protein-bound iodine. In addition, he carried out detailed studies of the mechanisms of thyroxine degradation. Robert H. Gibbs, M.D. (Chief, Medical Service, Jack C. Montgomery VAMC, Muskogee, OK) collaborated on a number of these studies.

The subsequent investigators carried out research in a broad gamut of endocrine diseases. Surprisingly, none of these individuals were involved in basic studies of diabetes.

J. Earl White, M.D. studied the lipolytic action of various hormones on adipose tissue. In addition, he defined the clinical course of familial hypophosphatemia.

Samuel J. Friedberg, M.D. studied the biochemistry of fatty acid metabolism in a variety of clinical pathologic situations. He directed the Cooperative Lipid Laboratory for several years.

Roger W. Turkington, M.D. carried out extensive studies of factors which control mammary gland development and function.

Marc K. Drezner, M.D. (Chief, Endocrinology, DUMC) evaluated the effects on bone metabolism of a number of hormonal and mineral factors.

Jerome M. Feldman, M.D. performed extensive studies of the natural history of a variety of neuro-endocrine tumors, including carcinoid and pheochromocytoma. He developed a number of novel approaches to the diagnosis and care of patients with these diseases.

Of these seven investigators, three had long-term academic careers, one remaining at DUMC. Approximately 505 manuscripts were authored or co-authored by them.

Medicine/Gastroenterology

The scope of the outstanding and long-term research effort in Gastroenterology has encompassed a wide range of fundamental studies of the pathophysiology and function of the gastrointestinal tract, the hepatobiliary system and the pancreas.

Malcolm P. Tyor, M.D. (Chief, Gastroenterology, DUMC) initiated studies related to ammonia metabolism. He defined the relationship between ammonia levels and the degree of hepatic encephalopathy in patients with severe liver disease.

Eugene E. Owen, M.D. carried out basic studies of ammonia metabolism and production in both the liver and kidney.

Paul D. Webster, III, M.D. (Chairman, Department of Medicine, Medical College of Georgia) carried out an evaluation of pancreatic RNA and amylase synthesis in response to stimulation by methacholine.

Steven H. Quarfordt, M.D. studied a number of aspects of cholesterol metabolism in liver disease. He developed an elaborate kinetic analysis for cholesterol metabolism. His primary contribution was the original isolation of apolipoprotein E. In addition, he directed the Cooperative Lipid Laboratory for a number of years.

William O. Dobbins, III, M.D. (Chief, Medicine Service, DVA) carried out extensive studies of histopathology in the gastrointestinal tract using electron microscopy. He had a special interest in inflammatory bowel disease and in Whipple's disease.

Charles M. Mansbach, II, M.D. (Chief, Gastroenterology, University of Tennessee Health Sciences Center) described the geographical location of the most important enzymes in complex lipid synthesis in the intestine. He discovered a unique regulatory site for the control of phosphatidylcholine biosynthesis.

Ian L. Taylor, M.D., Ph.D. (Dean, College of Medicine, SUNY Downstate Medical Center) transferred his research laboratory from the VA Hospital, Sepulveda, CA. His primary area of interest was the gastrointestinal hormone peptide YY (PYY) and its family of related peptides. He became a leading authority on the role of PYY in the gastrointestinal tract. Peter J. Mannon, M.D. continued this area of investigation productively for several years.

Stephen R. Vigna, Ph.D.* focuses his research on the gastrointestinal peptide bombesin and the characterization of its receptors. He extended this research into the gastrointestinal peptides of the enteric nervous system.

Rodger A. Liddle, M.D.* (Chief, Gastroenterology, DUMC) developed a unique assay for measuring blood levels of the satiety hormone, cholecystokinin and established the physiologic role of cholecystokinin as a regulator of gall bladder contraction, gastric emptying and insulin secretion and satiety. This work led to advanced studies on the neurohormonal regulation of the pancreas and the pathogenesis of pancreatitis.

Jonathan A. Cohn, M.D.* characterized the epithelial chloride transporter known as cystic fibrosis transmembrane regulator (CFTR) that is defective in cystic fibrosis. He successfully generated sensitive and specific antibodies against human CFTR. Also, he demonstrated that mutations in CFTR predisposed patients to chronic pancreatitis.

Toan D. Nguyen, M.D. studied the vasoactive intestinal peptide (VIP) and its family of related peptides. These studies focused on the signal transduction pathways downstream from G-protein coupled receptor binding.

Dawn T. Provenzale, M.D., M.P.H.* established a research program in gastroenterology outcomes research. She was instrumental in creating a method to obtain quality of life measurements for patients with esophageal dysphasia, esophageal cancer and colon cancer. In addition, she established guidelines for colon cancer surveillance.

This group of highly productive investigators authored or co-authored approximately 885 scientific publications. Of the 13 investigators listed, all but one had a predominant academic career, with six remaining at DUMC.

Medicine/General Medicine

Although General Medicine has existed as a separate division at DUMC and the DVA for only the past two and one-half decades, a large number of outstanding investigators have developed a comprehensive research program under the aegis of HSR&D. In fact, they are, by far, the largest research group at the DVA.

John R. Feussner, M.D., M.P.H. (Chairman, Department of Medicine, Medical University of South Carolina), studied the long-term outcomes of patients with different chronic diseases who were subjected to different treatment modalities. These studies concentrated on diseases which specifically affect the Veteran population. He was able to amplify this research as the Chief, Research and Development Officer, Department of Veterans Affairs.

Ramon Velez, M.D., M.P.H. (Head, General Internal Medicine and Gerontology, Wake Forest School of Medicine) evaluated a number of strategies for screening breast and cervical cancer and diabetic retinopathy.

Eugene Z. Oddone, M.D., M.H.S.* (Chief, General Medicine, DUMC and Director, Center for Health Sciences Research in Primary Care, DVA) studied the effects of access to care on outcomes of care for Veterans with chronic medical illnesses. He tests interventions designed to enhance access to care outside of the clinic by using novel technologies.

David B. Matchar, M.D., M.H.S.* (Director, Center for Clinical Health Policy, DUMC) applies complex mathematical models to common health care problems such as stroke care, chronic kidney disease and headache in an attempt to underscore how improvements in treatment and quality of care could simultaneously enhance patients' lives and achieve cost-effectiveness. He implements a number of analyses for the Evidence Based Practice Center funded by the Agency for Healthcare Quality and Research.

David L. Simel, M.D.* (ACOS, Ambulatory Care, DVA) carried out a number of clinical studies which crystallized the use of a number of modalities in the physical examination. The goal of his efforts is to positively influence the clinical care of Veterans as well as improve bedside teaching.

Ronnie D. Horner, Ph.D. (Director, Health Services Research, University of Cincinnati Medical School) studied the epidemiology of neurodegenerative diseases including stroke and amyelotrophic lateral sclerosis (ALS). His novel work with Persian Gulf War Veterans established a link between deployment to the Persian Gulf and ALS, thereby convincing the VA to offer a new disability category.

Hayden B. Bosworth, Ph.D.* focuses on implementing self-management interventions to improve long-term outcomes among individuals with chronic diseases, including hypertension, diabetes and hyperlipidemia. Currently, he is focusing on implementing these interventions into the Veteran population.

Lori A. Bastian, M.D., M.P.H.* is the original director of the women's health program at the DVA. She conducts research in a variety of issues in women's health and smoking cessation.

Rowena J. Dolor, M.D., M.H.S.* conducts clinical and outcomes research within Veteran and community-based primary care practices. She is a site investigator and executive committee member on a VA cooperative study, assessing the effectiveness of home prothrombin monitoring in Veterans.

David Edelman, M.D., M.H.S.* studies the clinical epidemiology of diabetes mellitus and its complications, and also studies the effectiveness of primary care interventions to improve diabetes outcomes. His studies of the outcomes of diabetes screening and group medical visits for patients with diabetes had immediate impact on the nearly one million VA patients with diabetes.

Karen E. Steinhauser, Ph.D.* has conducted studies to understand patient, family and provider perspectives on what is important at the end of life. She has, and is, developing tools to assess quality of that experience for patients and families and has implemented intervention studies designed to improve symptoms and quality of life for patients with advanced serious illness.

James A. Tulsky, M.D.* has studied physician-patient communication at the end of life and the experiences of dying patients. Projects have included: a multi-site study of audiotaped discussions between physicians and patients about advance directives; a series of studies that have helped define the attributes of a "good dying" culminating in the development of the QUAL-E, a measure of quality of life at the end of life, a study of 700 conversations between oncologists and patients with advanced cancer and a randomized, controlled trial of an intervention to improve communication, and a longitudinal cohort study of the functional, psychosocial, and spiritual trajectories of patients with advanced illness and their caregivers.

Morris Weinberger, Ph.D. (Director, Program on Health Outcomes, Department of Health Policy and Administration, University of North Carolina) uses randomized trials to evaluate strategies designed to improve the process and outcomes of care. His research generally targets elderly patients with chronic disease, such as those receiving care at the DVA.

John D. Whited, M.D., M.H.S.* has devoted much of his research efforts to the study of telemedicine, in particular teledermatology and teleophthalmology. His studies have evaluated a wide range of health services aspects of telemedicine implementation, including diagnostic reliability and accuracy, economic analyses, patient and provider satisfaction, and clinical outcomes.

John W. Williams, Jr., M.D.* has focused on problems at the interface between primary care and other disciplines. His research has helped to identify better approaches to diagnosing and treatment of acute sinusitis and the management of depression in primary care settings. Most of his research has been focused specifically on Veterans.

William S. Yancy, Jr., M.D., M.H.S.* studies the effects of dietary carbohydrate restriction on disorders commonly found in the Veteran population, specifically, obesity, diabetes, and cardiovascular disease. Also, he examines the relationships among obesity, health care utilization, and health outcomes.

Carol S. Hammond, Ph.D.* studies the aspects of osteoporosis as well as measures of rehabilitation and mobility aids on functional outcomes.

Kelli L.D. Allen, Ph.D.* studies self management interventions in patients with osteoarthritis.

Corrine I. Voils, Ph.D.* studies a number of modalities to lower LDL cholesterol with a particular interest on patient spouse interactions.

Of these 19 investigators, all have had a long-term academic career with 15 remaining at DUMC. They authored or co-authored approximately 1145 manuscripts.

Medicine/Geriatrics

Although only in existence for the past two decades, under the guidance of Harvey J. Cohen, M.D., research in Geriatrics has undergone phenomenal growth and productivity.

Harvey J. Cohen, M.D.* (Chairman, Department of Medicine, DUMC) initiated research which involved lymphocyte physiology and contributed to an understanding of membrane dynamics in normal and immunoproliferation disorders. Subsequently, his work described some of the features of immunosenescence. He was among the first to investigate the characteristics of cancer and immunoproliferative disorders in the elderly and the use of geriatric assessment in frail elders and those with cancer.

Lina M. Obeid, M.D. focused on the study of signal transduction pathways in cellular senescence and programmed cell death, two important models of growth arrest. Two areas of research were undertaken: 1) delineating the role of the newly discovered sphingomyelin cycle in cellular senescence and apoptosis, 2) investigating the role of the well-characterized phospholipid signaling pathways in cellular senescence.

Stephanie A. Studenski, M.D., M.P.H., directed her research efforts in rehabilitation related areas, such as risk factors and mechanisms of instability in the elderly. She also participated in clinical research projects assessing muscular skeletal problems of the elderly. The goal of her research was to reduce the consequences of falls, specifically injuries, which further reduce mobility and increase social isolation.

Kenneth W. Lyles, M.D.* heads the bone and fracture group and carried out a number of studies on two diseases that have a significant impact upon older Veterans: 1) osteoporosis and osteoporotic fractures and 2) Paget's disease of the bone. In the former category, it was found that following a hip fracture, subsequent clinical fractures are quite common and have marked negative impact on health. In Paget's disease, agents which improve the physical component scores in patients have been developed.

Kenneth E. Schmader, M.D.* studies the epidemiology of herpes zoster, evaluating two new risk factors: psychological stress and race. Dr. Schmader also examined the accuracy of self-reports of herpes zoster and found that a positive self-report has high positive predictive value and a negative self-report has a very high negative predictive value compared to physician diagnosis. Dr. Schmader is a lead investigator in the landmark VA Cooperative Study: Trial of Varicella Vaccine for the Prevention of Herpes Zoster and Its Complications, commonly known as the Shingles Prevention Study. The vaccine reduced the burden of illness due to herpes zoster by 61.1 percent, reduced the incidence of postherpetic neuralgia by 66.5 percent, and reduced the incidence of herpes zoster by 51.3 percent. Thus, the vaccine has the potential to reduce the incidence of herpes zoster by one half and postherpetic neuralgia by two-thirds in older Veterans.

Miriam C. Morey, Ph.D.* developed an exercise and health promotion clinical demonstration program that became the catalyst for studies of aging and exercise. Over the past two decades, Dr. Morey carried out a variety of longitudinal studies examining the impact of regular exercise on outcomes related to cardiovascular risk factors, physical function, adherence and mortality. This work involved a variety of clinical trials aimed at increasing physical functioning and decreasing disability in older Veterans with multiple chronic conditions. In addition, Dr. Morey has collaborated with the staff of other Veterans Affairs Medical Centers in implementing research in primary care and research settings such as home-based tele-care.

Helen M. Hoenig, M.D., M.P.H.* facilitated a highly collaborative rehabilitation outcomes research program which measured quality of care and impact of mobility on functional outcomes.

Harold G. Koenig, M.D., M.H.S.* studies depression in the medically ill elderly emphasizing the role of religion on health and aging (with an emphasis on religious coping and depression). He has made important observations regarding the association of religious participation and improved health.

Cathleen S. Colon-Emeric, M.D., M.H.S.* carries out clinical trials and health services interventions to decrease fracture rates in older adults, and to improve the quality of care in skilled nursing facilities. Results have included the development of nursing-home specific fracture risk assessment tools, quality improvement interventions for falls and osteoporosis, computerized order entry algorithms promoting guideline-recommended care for geriatric syndromes in nursing facilities, and a large multinational trial identifying a once-yearly drug that reduces the risk of further fractures in hip fracture patients.

Elizabeth C. Clipp, Ph.D.* concentrated her research efforts in four interrelated areas: a) the effects of military participation on the health and well-being of aging Veterans; b) the impact of informal caregiving on families in the context of progressive chronic illness, e.g., dementia; c) the development of clinically related methods for better understanding the dynamics of health in later life; and d) the integration of psychosocial and clinical issues in the assessment and care of elderly patients with cancer.

Gregory A. Taylor, Ph.D.* uses biochemical, cell biological, and mouse gene targeting approaches to study mechanisms of innate resistance to infection, particularly those active against infections prevalent in the elderly. He has identified a family of proteins (IRG proteins, or Immunity-Related GTPases) that are essential for innate resistance to many intracellular bacteria and protozoa, including *Mycobacterium tuberculosis*, *Salmonella typhimurium*, and *Toxoplasma gondii*. He has determined that IRG proteins function by regulating survival of pathogens in host cells, such as macrophages, with individual IRG proteins having distinct functions at both the cellular and physiological level.

Eleanor S. McConnell, Ph.D.* focuses on strengthening the scientific understanding of how best to provide bedside nursing care for older adults with cognitive impairment. Her contributions have been in three key areas: (1) understanding the interaction between physical mobility and cognitive impairment, using large clinical data sets, and through the conduct of clinical studies; (2) testing interventions that may slow the rate of decline in physical function among very frail older adults; and (3) understanding factors that accelerate the implementation of evidence based practices in nursing care.

Of these 12 investigators, all have had academic careers with ten remaining at DUMC. Approximately 970 manuscripts were authored or co-authored by these investigators.

Medicine/Hematology and Medical Oncology

The Hematology and Medical Oncology Section has been populated by a number of outstanding physician scientists who carried out the dual role of research and clinical care. Three of these served as Chief, Medical Service, DVA.

John Laszlo, M.D. (Vice President for Research, American Cancer Society) studied the pathogenesis and treatment of human leukemia, and myloprolific diseases as well as the pharmacology of anti-neoplastic drugs and the control of drug-induced nausea and vomiting.

William B. Kremer, M.D. investigated the efficacy of a variety of anti-leukemia drugs in patients.

J. Brice Weinberg, M.D.* (ACOS for Research and Development, DVA) focused on various aspects of phagocyte biology, specifically monocytes and macrophages and the host resistance to infection in patients with leukemia or inflamation. This work involved a number of different studies of the role of nitric oxide in disease processes including leukemia, rheumatoid arthritis, osteoarthritis, lupus erythematosus and malaria. In addition, these studies have found that nitric oxide can induce gene expression and differentiation of acute leukemia cells and normal blood forming cells.

Gerald L. Logue, M.D. (Chief, Hematology, State University of Buffalo Medical School) studied immunohematology with special expertise in autoimmune neutropenia.

Roger J. Kurlander, M.D. studied the immunology of monocytes and macrophage function investigating the immune response to foreign antigens and infections.

Jeffrey E. Crawford, M.D. (Chief, Medical Oncology, DUMC) studied the proteins in patients with gammopathies as well as the biology of lymphocytic neoplasms. In addition, he defined the use of hematopoietic growth factors in the supportive treatment of patients with cancer.

Robert L. Fine, M.D. studied cancer pharmacology including the cellular effects of a variety of agents used in the therapy of pancreatic cancer.

Paul J. Shami, M.D. studied the control of normal and leukemic hematopoieses with the goal to develop drugs for the treatment of leukemia.

Gerold Bepler, M.D., Ph.D. (Chief, Thoracic Oncology, University of South Florida) studied the basic biology of the pathogenesis of lung cancer emphasizing the development of new strategies for treatment.

Jared Gollob, M.D.* studies molecular signaling pathways in targeted immunotherapy for urologic cancer and melanoma.

Michael J. Kelley, M.D.* studies the molecular biology of cancer especially as it relates to lung cancer, chordoma and inherited platelet abnormalities. In addition, he carries out a number of clinical trials in the therapy of lung cancer.

Of these 11 investigators, nine have had long-term careers in academic medicine with four remaining at DUMC. These investigators authored or co-authored approximately 987 manuscripts.

Medicine/Infectious Diseases

In addition to their long-term vital clinical roles, which include infection surveillance and control, these investigators have made notable contributions to the understanding of the pathophysiology of infection both at a national and international level.

Richard V. McCloskey, M.D. studied the relationship between several antibiotics and renal function, specifically defining the effects of renal failure on serum levels of antibiotics.

John D. Hamilton, M.D.* (Chief, Infectious Diseases, DUMC) has had a long-time and very productive research interest in virology. Specifically, he has carried out in-depth studies of viral hepatitis, the human immunodeficiency virus and cytomegalovirus. Dr. Hamilton also was designated as the principal investigator for the VA-based AIDS Research Network.

Kenneth E. Wilson, M.D.* in collaboration with Ronald C. Greene, Ph.D. developed a number of probes to directly detect and quantify bacteria in the colon. Also, he was the first to identify Tropheryma whippelii, the probable cause of Whipple's disease. In addition, he was asked by the intelligence community to help develop ways to identify biological warfare agents by molecular means.

Charles van der Horst, M.D. carried out HIV clinical research focusing primarily on the neurocognitive effects of high viral loads as well as other co-infections.

Richard Frothingham, M.D.* studies the pathophysiology of Mycobacterium avium. The ultimate goal of this investigation is the development of TB vaccines which are effective in adults. Recently, Drs. Frothingham and Wilson have teamed together to develop a research program at the DVA which has as its goal the development of drugs, vaccines and diagnostics for emerging infections and biodefense.

Carol D. Hamilton, M.D.* studies the effects of human immunodeficiency virus on the course of other infectious diseases. These studies were carried out primarily in Tanzanian patients.

Mary E. Klotman, M.D. (Chief, Infectious Diseases, Mt. Sinai Medical School) studied the pathophysiology of cytomegalovirus renal allograths in both murine and human subjects. In addition, she studied a variety of cellular responses to HIV-1 infection.

Christopher W. Woods, M.D.* utilizes the electronic medical record of the VA Health System to perform translational research in emerging pathogens, novel diagnostics, and resistant nosocomial organisms. In particular, his epidemiological investigations of the emergence of novel strains of *Clostridium difficile* in the hospital and in the community, using a combination of automated surveillance and molecular techniques, has become a model for infection control programs in the VA. Dr. Woods also maintains international programs to perform sentinel surveillance for emerging infections in the developing world.

Of these eight investigators, seven have continued in a long-term academic career with five remaining at DUMC. One investigator has had a distinguished career in industry. Approximately 531 publications have been authored or co-authored by these individuals.

Medicine/Nephrology

In addition to their primary function of developing and maintaining an extensive renal dialysis program, the Nephrology group at the DVA fostered a number of outstanding physician scientists who have had a sustained output of outstanding research.

Roscoe R. Robinson, M.D. (Vice Chancellor for Health Affairs, Vanderbilt University Medical Center) characterized the metabolism and release of ammonia by the kidney. In most of these studies, he collaborated with Eugene E. Owen, M.D. (Gastroenterology). In addition, Dr. Robinson initiated an extensive series of studies which define the pathophysiology of orthostatic proteinuria.

Cleaves M. Bennett, M.D. studied control mechanisms of filtration in the distal nephron.

William E. Yarger, M.D.* (Chief, Medicine Service, DVA) studied the pathophysiology of renal obstruction, hyperuricemic renal disease and gentamicin nephrotoxicity. Also, he defined the role of both prostaglandins and arachidonic acid metabolites in regulating renal blood flow.

Robert A. Gutman, M.D. used Xenon measurements to evaluate renal blood flow in pathological circumstances such as acute renal failure.

Peter C. Brazy, M.D. (Chief, Nephrology, Wisconsin Medical School) carried out extensive studies on the metabolism of transport in renal tubules.

Laura P. Svetkey, M.D. evaluated a number of strategies for the diagnosis of renal vascular hypertension and genetics of salt-sensitivity in African Americans. In addition, she studied the efficacy of a number of antihypertensive regimens.

William W. Stead, M.D. (Associate Vice Chancellor for Health Affairs and Chief Information Officer, Vanderbilt University

Medical Center) developed an electronic medical record. His first program, TMR (The Medical Record), was initially tested in the DVA Renal Clinic and was later used in a number of outpatient clinics.

Robert H. Harris, Jr., M.D. investigated the pathophysiology of renal obstruction. He carried out a series of studies measuring natriuretic factors in urine which were found in obstructive neuropathy.

Thomas M. Coffman, M.D.* (Chief, Nephrology, DUMC) evaluates kidney inflammation, transplant rejection and the renal angiotensin system using genetically engineered mice.

Paul E. Klotman, M.D. (Chairman, Department of Medicine, Mount Sinai Medical School, NY) studied gentamicin nephrotoxcicity and thromboxane in renal disease and HIV nephropathy.

John R. Raymond, Sr., M.D. (Vice President for Academic Affairs and Provost, Medical University of South Carolina) studied g-protein coupled receptors with a focus on the serotonin receptor.

Roslyn B. Mannon, M.D. studied the role of major incompatibility antigens in chronic renal transplant rejection.

Robert F. Spurney, M.D.* evaluates molecular signaling in the kidney focusing on thromboxane and parathyroid hormone receptors.

Steven D. Crowley, M.D.* studies the role of angiotensin receptors in the kidney which control blood pressure in both normal physiology and in hypertension.

Mary H. Foster, M.D.* studies B cell tolerance in basement membranes as it applies to autoimmune nephritis.

Thu H. Le, M.D.* evaluates genetic susceptibility in chronic kidney disease.

Fourteen of these 16 investigators pursued a long-term career in academic medicine with seven remaining at DUMC. They authored or co-authored approximately 964 scientific manuscripts.

Medicine/Neurology

Research in the pathophysiology of the nervous system has had a high profile role at the DVA since its inception. The scope of the investigations has produced a number of unique findings defining the pathophysiology of the nervous system in health and disease.

Albert Heyman, M.D. studied a number of factors which control the cerebral circulation during a variety of physiologic and pathologic conditions. In addition, he developed a long-term interest in defining the natural history of stroke and other cerebral diseases, specifically Alzheimer's disease.

Antonio V. Delgado-Escueta, M.D. studied the pathogenesis of epilepsy using the freeze lesion model in the cat. He was responsible for developing the Epilepsy Center at the DVA.

Saul M. Schanberg, M.D. studied the roles of a variety of receptors in the metabolism and function of the brain.

James O. McNamara, M.D. (Chairman, Department of Neurobiology, DUMC) carried out ground-breaking studies in both the human and in animal models to define the pathophysiology and treatment of epilepsy. Cheolsu Shin, M.D. collaborated with Dr. McNamara in many of these studies.

James N. Davis, M.D. (Chairman, Department of Neurology, SUNY at Stony Brook) studied the role of receptors in the brain. In addition, he initiated both basic and clinical research in the natural history of stoke. This work led to the development of a Stroke Center at the DVA.

Wilkie A. Wilson, Ph.D.* studies the electrophysiology of neuroplasticity in the central nervous system with particular emphasis on the pathology of neuroplasticity as it relates to the genesis and expression of epilepsy, amnestic disorders and addictive processes. For several years, Andrew C. Bragdon, M.D. collaborated in a number of these investigations.

Larry B. Goldstein, M.D.* defines the immediate repair response of the brain following stroke and its modification by various pharmacologic modalities. In addition, he has catalogued the long-term outcomes of patients with stroke.

David A. Hosford, M.D., Ph.D. studied the role GABAA and GABAB receptors in the development of generalized seizures using a combination of anatomical and electrophysiologic techniques. He studied mechanisms which produce absence seizures. In addition, he characterized the genetics of these seizures.

Donald E. Schmechel, M.D.* carried out detailed studies of neuronal receptors in primates. His primary area of interest was in the study of animal models which mimic Alzheimer's disease.

Richard S. Bedlack, M.D., Ph.D.* is a national thought leader in research on Veterans with amyotrophic lateral sclerosis (ALS). He is an integral part of a large registry which contains demographic and clinical information for more than 2,000 Veterans who have been diagnosed as having ALS. These data are being used to characterize the natural history of this disease and to analyze factors which might impact this, including military service and service in different specific conflicts. He is involved in a multicenter trial of sodium phenylbutyrate to determine if this drug, in a tolerable dose, alters transcription and slows progression in patients with ALS. His latest endeavor is a study of an exciting "brain-computer interface" that may help restore communication to Veterans with late state ALS.

Of these 12 investigators, 11 have pursued a long-term academic career with seven remaining at DUMC. In addition, one individual has an investigative career in industry. Approximately 1150 manuscripts were authored or co-authored by these individuals.

Medicine/Pulmonary

Pulmonary Research at the DVA can be categorized into five main areas: 1) cardio-pulmonary interactions, 2) pulmonary development, anatomy and pathology, 3) oxidative stress and oxidative injury 4) surfactant metabolism and function and 5) pulmonary inflammation, injury and repair. This research has emphasized the pathogensis of several important chronic lung diseases such as chronic bronchitis, emphysema, and several rare lung diseases such as byssinosis, asbestos and pulmonary alveolar proteinosis.

Shortly after the DVA opened, Herbert O. Sieker, M.D. (Chief, Pulmonary, DUMC) began clinical studies of cardiopulmonary interactions. This work led to one of the first descriptions of the pickwickian syndrome. In addition, Dr. Sieker carried out extensive studies of the mechanisms of sleep apnea.

Herbert A. Saltzman, M.D. carried out a number of studies involving pulmonary gas exchange. These led to a long-term interest in the pathophysiology of hyperbaria and the use of this modality in the treatment of a variety of disease processes.

Juan Ramirez, M.D. measured the nature and origin of alveolar lipid in pulmonary alveolar proteinosis, asthma and chronic bronchitis. Donald J. Massaro, M.D. studied surfactant metabolism at the DVA near the beginning of his long and illustrious career in biomedical research.

William S. Lynn, M.D., who previously had studied phospholipids, turned his full-time research activities to the biology of glycoproteins and fatty acids in the lung during macromolecular damage. In addition, he studied protein-lipid oxidation and sulfhydryl oxidation during pulmonary inflammation.

Kaye H. Kilburn, M.D. (Chief, Medicine Service, DVA) and Philip C. Pratt, M.D. (Pathology) studied the pathogenesis and pathologic findings of respiratory failure including alveolar lung damage and goblet cell metaplasia. Drs. Kilburn and Pratt also conducted work on the effects of exposure to nitrogen dioxide on pulmonary ultrastructure compliance and the surfactant system. In addition, they studied exposure to cotton dust, papain-induced emphysema and the biological effects of cigarette smoking on the pathogenesis of pulmonary disease.

During the past two decades, there were three independent pulmonary investigators at the DVA: Stephen L. Young, M.D.* (ACOS for Research and Development, DVA), Lyn A. Thet, M.D. and Claude A. Piantadosi, M.D.* Dr. Thet's interests were primarily in postneumonectomy lung growth and lung repair after acute lung injury, especially hyperoxia and other oxidant injury mechanisms such as paraquat. Dr. Young concentrated his efforts on understanding surfactant kinetics and its relationship to biochemical and morphometric endpoints in acute lung injury. Also, he studied the efficacy of natural and artificial surfactants to protect against acute lung injury in primates.

Dr. Piantadosi, who had a long-term interest in hyperbaric medicine, studied the effects of hypoxia and ischemia on the brain, lung and heart mitochondria, focusing more recently on understanding the important role of oxidative and nitrosative stress in acute lung injury and multi-organ failure in sepsis—a major cause of death in the Veteran population over age 55. Dr. Piantadosi recently has discovered that inflammation not only leads to oxidative mitochondrial damage, especially to mitochondria DNA, but also stimulates mitochondria biogenesis. Currently, Dr. Piantadosi continues his work focusing on a basic level of biochemical signaling and molecular toxicity of reactive oxygen and nitrogen species. In these studies, he collaborates with Karen E. Welty-Wolf, M.D.* and Timothy J. McMahon, M.D., Ph.D.*

David A. Schwartz, M.D., M.P.H.* (Chief, Pulmonary and Critical Care, DUMC) transferred his very productive research program from the University of Iowa. His research is focused on the identification of genetic variation in the response to inhaled toxins. Julia K. Walker, Ph.D.* collaborated in a number of these investigations.

Twelve of these 13 investigators have had long-term academic careers with nine remaining at DUMC. Approximately 1318 manuscripts were authored or co-authored by these individuals.

Medicine/Rheumatology and Immunology

William P. Deiss, M.D. (Chairman, Department of Medicine, UT Galveston) studied the polysaccharide components of mucoprotein in both bone and valvular tissue. In addition, he defined the effects of thyrotropin on serum protein-bound iodine.

David S. Pisetsky, M.D.* (Chief, Rheumatology, DUMC) carried out an extensive series of studies defining the antibody recognition of DNA in normal and aberrant immunity. He found that patients with systemic lupus erythematosus had antibodies broadly reactive with all DNA, whereas normal people had antibodies that bound selectively to bacterial DNA. Subsequently, Dr. Pisetsky showed that bacterial DNA can stimulate B cell activation, providing important evidence for the role of foreign DNA in innate immunity. More recently, Dr. Pisetsky's research has involved evaluating extracellular DNA as a marker of cell death in conditions such as shock and malignancy. For his work on the immune properties of DNA, Dr. Pisetsky received the Howley Prize from the Arthritis Foundation.

Gary S. Gilkeson, M.D. carried out a series of in-depth studies characterizing anti-DNA antibodies in mice under a variety of pathologic situations which includes spontaneous murine autoimmune disease.

These three investigators have continued long-term academic careers with one remaining at DUMC. Approximately 375 manuscripts have been authored or co-authored by these three individuals.

Mental Health

The Mental Health Service Line (formerly Psychiatry Service) has had an integral role in the research endeavors of the DVA throughout the past five decades. The scope of this outstanding research has varied from basic electrophysiology to clinical studies of the deleterious effects of traumatic stress.

William P. Wilson, M.D. utilized electroencephalography to define the effects of a variety of physiologic and pathologic conditions on cerebral function. He specifically quantitated the effects of increased intracranial pressure as well as elevated levels of ammonia in blood.

William W.K. Zung, M.D. carried out a number of in-depth studies in defining depression. One of the most widely utilized scales to quantitate depression was developed by Dr. Zung.

Herbert F. Crovitz, Ph.D. studied the cognitive effects of electroconvulsive therapy. He also studied the pathophysiology of visual perception.

Richard D. Weiner, M.D., Ph.D.* (Chief, Mental Health Service Line, DVA) conducted research on the optimization of electroconvulsive therapy including the reduction of cognitive sequela and EEG changes following this treatment modality.

H. Scott Swartzwelder, Ph.D.* studies the effects of alcohol on the central nervous system. He is noted primarily for describing the effects of alcohol on the adolescent brain as compared to the adult brain. His work is based on electrophysiological and behavioral modalities.

W. Edward Fann, M.D. studied the pharmacology of a variety of psychotrophic drugs. In addition, he carried out extensive studies of tardive dyskinesia.

Jed E. Rose, Ph.D.* performed extensive studies in the neurobiology of nicotine dependence and smoking cessation strategies.
He conducted neuroimaging and genetic studies related to nicotine dependence.

Christine E. Marx, M.D.* initiated a series of ongoing investigations focusing on neuroactive steroids utilizing a high sensitive
and specific mass spectrometry-based method. She also conducts
clinical trials in patients with schizophrenia and post traumatic
stress disorder.

Jack D. Edinger, Ph.D.* studies the pathophysiology of sleep.
He has conducted extensive research focusing on effective non
pharmacological interventions for insomnia.

Keith G. Meador, M.D., M.P.H., Th.M.* studies the interface between both spirituality and religion and mental disorders. He also
studies severe mental illness and directs the inpatient psychiatry unit.

Lawrence Dunn, M.D. studied the treatment and pathophysiology of schizophrenia and was involved in multiple pivotal clinical trials focusing on psychotic disorders.

Gregory McCarthy, Ph.D.* is a leader in functional neuroimaging correlates of cognition. He was the original Director of the
Mid-Atlantic Mental Illness Research Education and Clinical Center. (MIRECC).

The MIRECC is organized as a translational medicine center in
which the overarching goal is the clinical assessment and treatment
of post-deployment mental illness. The MIRECC focuses on the
following aims:

1) To determine whether early intervention in post-deployment mental health is effective in forestalling the development or decreasing the severity of post-deployment
   mental illness.
2) To determine what neuroimaging, genetic, neurocognitive, or other characteristics predict the development of
   post-deployment mental illness.
3) To assess the longitudinal course of post-deployment
   mental illness.

Studies as to the pathogenesis, natural history and treatment of
patients with post traumatic stress disorders (PTSD) with a pri-

mary interest in Vietnam combat Veterans, has been a major focus of the research carried out by the Center.

John A. Fairbank, Ph.D.* is the new Director of the MIRECC. He is an expert in research on traumatic stress in both Veterans and non-Veterans, primarily from a health services standpoint.

Harold S. Kudler, M.D.* studies PTSD and has served as the Co-Director for the Clinical Component of the Mid-Atlantic Mental Illness, Research, Education and Clinical Center. He also has held regional and national mental health leadership roles within the Veterans Affairs Hospital System.

Marian I. Butterfield, M.D., M.P.H.* was an expert in PTSD in female Veterans. She also implemented a variety of mental health services projects involving recently deployed Veterans. In addition, she chaired the American Psychiatric Association Scientific Program Committee.

Jonathan R. Davidson, M.D. studied PTSD and other anxiety disorders. He was also an expert on complementary approaches to psychiatric disorders. He led seminal clinical trials in the area of PTSD.

Jean C. Beckham, Ph.D.* is an expert in the diagnosis and treatment of PTSD. She also does extensive research in the area of nicotine dependence and PTSD.

Patrick S. Calhoun, Ph.D.* studies the effects of PTSD on Veterans and their families from a health service standpoint.

Michael A. Hertzberg, M.D.* conducts pharmacological clinical trials in Veterans with PTSD and has provided leadership in the PTSD Clinical Program at the DVA.

Loretta E. Braxton, Ph.D.* studied personality inventory profiles of Vietnam combat Veterans. She was also involved in nicotine cessation research.

Scott D. Moore, M.D., Ph.D.* is a leader in studies of the physiology of the amygdala. He studies PTSD, traumatic brain injury (TBI) and alcohol use disorders.

Of these 21 investigators, 20 have had a long-term academic career with 19 remaining at DUMC. These investigators together authored or co-authored approximately 1700 publications.

Ophthalmology

Diane L. Hatchell, Ph.D. utilized animal models of diabetic retinopathy to determine the vascular and ocular changes which occur before the development of clinically observable retinopathy. These studies demonstrated an increase in glycosylated proteins in the vitreous humor of diabetic rabbits. Treatment with aminoguanidine was shown to inhibit reactive oxygen species formation, lipid peroxidation and oxidant-induced apoptosis in ocular fluids and tissues. Retinal hypoxia was also demonstrated in early diabetic retinopathy and was correlated with endothelial cell death, leukocyte plugging of vessels and microaneurysms. All of these alterations potentially contribute to the development of microangiopathies.

Dr. Hatchell pursued a long-term academic career and authored or co-authored 84 manuscripts.

Pathology and Laboratory Medicine

In 1958, Wiley D. Forbus, M.D. (Chairman, Department of Pathology, DUMC) hired Joachim R. Sommer, M.D. to direct the autopsy service at the DVA. This position allowed Dr. Sommer adequate time to develop an outstanding research program which received continuous research funding from 1962 until the time of his retirement in 1998. Dr. Sommer was a productive investigator, studying the relationships between the structure and function in myocardial cells. Interestingly, Dr. Sommer, as is true with a number of DVA investigators, received his salary support from non-VA sources and thus, was a WOC (without compensation) physician during this entire period. In 1962, he became Chief of the Electron Microscopy Laboratory and in 1971 obtained support for a new program: Diagnostic Electron Microscopy. These facilities, later directed by Dr. Shelburne, provided state of the art morphological images for a number of research investigators as well as patient care. The capabilities of the facility were enhanced by James D. Crapo, M.D. (Chief, Pulmonary and Critical Care, DUMC) who was instrumental in obtaining funding for an additional electron microscope which he used to define lung morphology associated with hypoxic injury.

John D. Shelburne, M.D., Ph.D.* (Chief of Staff, DVA) as Director of the Electron Microscopy Laboratory studied microprobe analysis of xenobiotics. In addition, he collaborated with a number of investigators who used this laboratory for a wide variety of research endeavors.

Philip C. Pratt, M.D. collaborated with Dr. Kilburn (described in Medicine/Pulmonary), to define the morphologic consequences of lung injury. Dr. Pratt was especially interested in the effects of hyperoxic lung injury and was among the first to describe the pulmonary pathology on several patients who died after receiving

100% oxygen for prolonged periods of time. The pathology of asbestos related lung disease was defined by Victor L. Roggli, M.D. in collaboration with Dr. Pratt.

Fred P. Sanfilippo, M.D., Ph.D. (Dean, Health Sciences, The Ohio State University) studied a number of immunologic factors which were involved in enhancing the survival of transplanted tissue.

Robin T. Vollmer, M.D.* established that an intermediate variant of small cell lung cancer behaved like ordinary small cell lung cancer so that subsequent WHO classifications of lung cancer dropped this category. He established that tumor volume in prostate cancer is an important prognosticator. Although black men release more PSA per gram of tumor than white men, age or race related adjustment in PSA based algorithms used to decide when to biopsy the prostate were not found to be indicated. Dr. Vollmer introduced a measure of "information content", derived from laboratory tests, to demonstrate that current models for predicting outcomes in prostate cancer and malignant melanoma provide little prognostic information.

David N. Howell, M.D, Ph.D.* (Chief, Pathology and Laboratory Medicine Service, DVA) uses confocal microscopy to identify focal pathologic processes for subsequent ultrastructural study. A second area of interest is evaluating a number of factors which are involved in the pathophysiology of segmental glomerulosclerosis.

Maureane R. Hoffman, M.D., Ph.D.* studies blood coagulation. These investigations have resulted in a better understanding of the roles played by the intrinsic and extrinsic coagulation pathways in vivo.

Peter Zwadyk, M.D.* evaluated a number of technologies which were useful in the clinical microbiology laboratory. His major focus was the use of nucleic acid probes in the diagnosis of infectious diseases. In fact, this research led to the establishment of a nucleic acid diagnostic laboratory.

E. Ann LeFurgey, M.D.* studies the processes by which Leishmania maintain ionic homeostasis in different environmental milieus.

Of these ten investigators, all have had long-term academic careers with nine remaining at DUMC. They authored or co-authored approximately 723 manuscripts.

Radiology

William M. Thompson, M.D. (Chairman, Department of Radiology, University of Minnesota Medical School) collaborated with a number of investigators to develop a variety of imaging techniques as well as the use of transcathether electro-coagulation. His primary interest was directed at the hepatobiliary system which involved both basic and clinical investigation. Robert A. Halvorsen, Jr., M.D. collaborated in many of these studies. In addition, Dr. Thompson evaluated radiographic techniques to define end-stage gastrointestinal carcinoma. Dr. Thompson has had a very distinguished academic career.

Gregory McCarthy, Ph.D. employs functional magnetic resonance imaging along with other modalities to evaluate the processing of complex visual stimuli. In addition, he uses a similar technology to investigate the function of prefrontal cortex.

All of these investigators have had long-term academic careers, one remaining at DUMC. They authored or co-authored approximately 305 scientific manuscripts.

Surgery/General Surgery

There have been a number of investigators in the General Surgical Section who carried out the dual roles of clinical care and investigation at the DVA from its inception until the present. Raymond W. Postlethwait, M.D. (Chief of Staff, DVA) established a laboratory addressing studies of esophageal motility and reflux disease. Through his efforts, the DVA was awarded a Regional Referral Center for benign and malignant diseases of the human esophagus.

A research program which had a major impact on the DVA was directed by Hilliard F. Seigler, M.D.* Dr. Seigler, trained by D. Bernard Amos, M.D. in immunogenetics at DUMC, began his research activities in 1965. His laboratory was supported both by NIH and VA funds until 1995. In addition to outstanding research, the Clinical Immunology and Tissue Typing Laboratory had its origin in the laboratory run by Dr. Seigler. Thus, much of the basic work which supported the initial transplant program at DUMC had its origin in his research program.

Donald Silver, M.D. (Chairman, Department of Surgery, University of Missouri Medical Center) headed a productive laboratory studying clotting factors and pulmonary embolism.

Delford L. Stickel, M.D. (Chief of Staff, DVA) concentrated his research efforts in the area of renal transplantation, obtaining the initial support for the transplant program at the DVA.

R. Scott Jones, M.D. (Chairman, Department of Surgery, University of Virginia, Charlottesville) initiated a series of studies of biliary function. He was joined by William C. Meyers, M.D. (Chairman, Department of Surgery, Drexler University, College of Medicine) who expanded the research program to include bowel metabolism and the etiology and management of peptide ulcer disease.

Onyekwere E. Akwari, M.D. studied pancreatic function with specific interest in the role of fatty acids in stimulating pancreatic and islet cell function.

John P. Grant, M.D. studied the role of total parenteral nutrition (TPN) in malnourished patients following a major surgical procedure. The rates in major and infectious complications were evaluated. The data indicated that in severely malnourished patients, major complications were fewer. However, the infectious complications were similar, indicating that TPN should be limited to patients who are severely malnourished.

Theodore (Ted) N. Pappas, M.D.* (Chief, Surgery Service, DVA) characterized the role of substance P in human disease. In addition, in collaboration with Toku Takahashi, M.D., Ph.D.* the pathophysiology of chronic motility has been evaluated. Dr. Takahashi has defined the role of acupuncture in the treatment of functional gastrointestinal disorders.

Douglas S. Tyler, M.D.* (Chief, Surgery Service, DVA) carries out a number of clinical and basic studies to better define the appropriate treatment of patients with abdominal cancer with a major interest in carcinoma of the pancreas. Scott K. Pruitt, M.D., Ph.D.* has collaborated in these investigations.

All of these 12 investigators have pursued academic careers with nine remaining at DUMC. Approximately 1519 manuscripts were authored or co-authored by these physician scientists.

Surgery/Cardiothoracic Surgery

The research carried out by these investigators was instrumental in facilitating the development of a vibrant open heart surgery program at the DVA.

Marcus L. Dillon, M.D. carried out a number of studies to define the characteristics of a variety of different suture materials.

Andrew S. Wechsler, M.D. (Chairman, Department of Cardiothoracic Surgery, Drexler University College of Medicine) directed his research effort toward defining factors which influenced the outcome during cardiopulmonary bypass. These extensive studies defined the appropriate infusion solutions during bypass procedures.

These two investigators have had long-term academic careers. Approximately 354 manuscripts were authored or co-authored by them.

Surgery/Neurosurgery

The clinical and research program headed by Neurosurgery has had a long and productive history. Byron M. Bloor, M.D. (Chairman, Department of Neurosurgery, University of West Virginia) carried out a number of studies of direct intravascular pressure in the vasculature of the brain to define the factors which control cerebral perfusion.

George T. Tindall, M.D. (Chairman, Department of Neurosurgery, Emory University) employed an electromagnetic flow meter to measure internal carotid artery blood flow. These studies defined the effects of position, intracranial pressure and a number of pharmacologic agents in the regulation of cerebral blood flow in man.

Wesley A. Cook, Jr., M.D. developed an outstanding motor function physiology laboratory.

Dennis A. Turner, M.D.* focuses on aging research, stroke and a variety of factors which influence the efficacy of neural grafting. He collaborates with Roger D. Madison, Ph.D.* in studying regenerative research in the nervous system. In addition, Dr. Turner developed an interest in neuroprosthetics for enhancing nervous system function. Ashok K. Shetty, Ph.D.* also collaborates with Dr. Turner, studying neurofilament expression in hippocampal grafts.

All six investigators have had long-term academic careers with four remaining at DUMC. The investigators authored or co-authored approximately 599 manuscripts.

Surgery/Orthopaedics

James R. Urbaniak, M.D. (Chief, Orthopaedics, DUMC) carried out a number of studies utilizing microvascular surgery which led to the development of the technology to successfully replant traumatically amputated limbs. In fact, his research laboratory microscope was transported to the DUMC Operating Room and used in the historical replant of a thumb in a 16 year old patient. His research was, indeed, of ground breaking importance in the successful repair of traumatic injuries. In this regard, a comment from Dr. Urbaniak should be documented: "It is obvious that Duke would have never achieved the national reputation in replantation surgery and microvascular reconstruction without our laboratory experience and funding at the DVA."

John M. Harrelson, M.D. studied bone histomorphometry in patients with X-linked hypophosphatemia and in patients with renal osteodystrophy.

William E. Garrett, Jr., M.D., Ph.D. (Chairman, Department of Orthopaedics, University of North Carolina, Chapel Hill) carried out a number of studies to evaluate the factors involved in muscle and tendon responses to acute strain injury. This work formed the basis for his long-term involvement in the care of patients with sports related injuries.

These investigators have had long-term academic careers with three remaining at DUMC. They authored or co-authored approximately 404 scientific manuscripts.

Surgery/Urology

David F. Paulson, M.D. (Chief, Urology, DUMC) assisted by Robert A. Bonar, Ph.D. worked for a number of years to define the in vitro responses to viruses, carcinogens and chemotherapy agents of a variety of cells cultured from urogenital tissues.

Recently, Karl B. Thor, Ph.D.* and Paul C. Dolber, Ph.D.* developed a laboratory of neuro-urology. Their work encompasses studies of alterations in adrenergic signaling in an animal model of bladder outlet obstruction and the study of neural changes consequent to experimental nerve lesions. Recently, Dr. Dolber's work became centered on the treatment of experimentally induced spinal cord injury and examination of the mechanisms underlying lower urinary tract dysfunction in spinal cord injury.

Stephen J. Freedland, M.D.* studies prostate cancer epidemiology and outcomes emphasizing the association between obesity and prostate cancer.

All five of these investigators have had a long-term academic career at DUMC. They authored or co-authored approximately 463 manuscripts.

Summation

The research program at the DVA has been functional for slightly longer than five decades. During that time, 215 investigators have carried out independent funded research at this institution. Of these, 179 were physicians and 36 non physicians. As a general rule, the nature of research carried out by both groups of investigators was oriented toward a better understanding of human disease processes. Judged by the number of publications documented, the research productivity has been outstanding.

For the entire group, 197 (92%) pursued a long-term career in academic medicine. Of these, 161 were physicians and 36 non physicians. In the physician group, 14 had a predominant career in practice and 4 had a career in either the pharmaceutical or biomedical industry (Table I, Panel A). All but one of this practice group spent less than five years as a research investigator.

In evaluating these career choices, the fact must be considered that the period of research for 91 of these individuals is five years or less. Although the transfer to a non academic career of non physician scientists is essentially zero, a number of physicians who initially begin in academic medicine choose practice for their predominant career. Thus, the figure of 92% may be spuriously high over the long term. In a recently published study of the career choices of cardiologists having an academic career of at least five years in duration, 20% ultimately chose private practice[7]. This figure probably is the upper limit for the DVA physician investigators. Assuming that 20% of the 91 physicians do pursue a long-term non academic career, the figure of 92% would be reduced to 83%—still very impressive.

Several of the physician investigators obtained additional academic degrees. For example, 15 of the physicians held a Ph.D. degree and 16 either had a Master of Health Sciences (M.H.S.) or Master of Public Health (M.P.H.) degree.

Of those remaining in academic medicine, 138 (70%) had their predominant career at DUMC and 60 (30%) went to other academic institutions. (Table I, Panel A). Seventy of this group spent their entire academic career at the DVA. A number of these individuals held important administrative positions within the academic institutions as well as the VA system. Six high level administrative positions, i.e., Dean, Provost, or Chancellor were filled by this group. There were 24 academic departments and 28 academic divisions led by these investigators. Nine of these scientists held high level positions within the VA system and 23 functioned in a Service Chief position. These are documented in Table I, Panel B.

Fifty-nine individuals who spent their career in academic institutions other than DUMC are located in 24 different states. The regional distribution of these individuals is as follows: South 24, Midwest 12, Northeast 17 and West 6.

There are a number of individuals who spent a long period of time carrying out research at the DVA. Table II lists the names, department/division affiliation, and research interests of 33 scientists who functioned in a research capacity at the DVA for at least a 20-year period. Ninty-one scientists have carried out research at the DVA for a period between ten and twenty years. Their department affiliations are as follows: Anesthesiology 4, Basic Sciences 5, Medicine 49, Mental Health 9, Ophthalmology 1, Pathology and Laboratory Medicine 8, Radiology 1, and Surgery 14.

The DVA has been instrumental in providing a milieu whereby scientists could begin their independent investigative career. Of the 215 investigators, 164 began their research career at the DVA.

The DVA has been a major factor in supporting the research endeavors of physicians who made a major impact on the Clinical Services. In fact, one of the very attractive features of the VA system was the availability of research funds for physician scientists. Also of note, there are a number of outstanding Ph.D. scientists who have made contributions to the research endeavors. The ratio of M.D./Ph.D. scientists has remained relatively static during the recent past. For example, in 1992, 21% of the investigators were Ph.D. scientists and in 2005, this number was 20%.

The VA Cooperative Studies Program has been used by many investigators to foster their research programs. In 2005, ten Cooperative studies are being carried out at the DVA. Four of these studies are chaired by DVA investigators.

Current assessment of research at the DVA clearly indicates an impressive and productive group of investigators. Of the long-term investigators listed in Table II, 23 are still active research leaders. In 2005, there are 55 investigators carrying out independent research projects funded, at least in part, by the VA. In addition, 80 investigators funded from non VA sources are actively involved in the Research Program at the DVA. The nature of their research varies from basic studies of molecular mechanisms to in-depth studies of clinical disease processes. When one considers the very difficult environment which has existed during the past ten years regarding research funding, this is an impressive number of independent investigators.

By any criteria, the scientific community who have functioned at the DVA are a remarkable group of individuals. The proof that the DVA has been a fertile ground for fostering the early careers of outstanding investigators and academicians is clearly documented by their accomplishments. Their research has been at the forefront in defining disease processes and in enhancing the care of Veteran patients. One would be hard pressed to find an institution with a better record.

Table I

Panel A			Career Affiliations		
Investigators	DUMC	DVA	Other Academic	Industry	Non Academic
215	138	70	59	4	14

Column1 lists the total number of investigators meeting the criteria for inclusion in the text.

Columns 2, 4-6 list the affiliation of these investigators.

Column 3 lists the number of investigators who spent their entire research career at the DVA.

Panel B		Academic Positions			
*Dean †Associate Dean	Other	Dept Chairman Chief	Dept Division	VA Admin Chief	VA Service
*1/5 †0/1	3/6	5/19	19/10	7/2	22/2

Each column lists the number of academic positions which were held by the DVA investigators.

Columns 1–4 (the first number) indicates a position at DUMC; the second at another academic institution. In columns 5 and 6, the first number indicates the position at the DVA and the second, a position elsewhere. (Note that an individual investigator may have held more than one of these academic positions.)

Column 2 lists the director of a major academic program, e.g., a cancer center or a full-time major role in a national organization, e.g., the American Cancer Society.

Table II
Long-Term Investigators

Name	Department/Division	Research Interests
Clipp, Elizabeth C.*	Medicine/Geriatrics	Aging
Cobb, Frederick R.*	Medicine/Cardiology	Cardiovascular Physiology
Coffman, Thomas M.*	Medicine/Nephrology	Renal Pathophysiology
Cohen, Harvey J.*	Medicine/Geriatrics	Cell Signaling and Aging
Crovitz, Herbert F.	Mental Health	Electroconvulsive Therapy
Feldman, Jerome M.	Medicine/Endocrinology	Neuroendocrine Tumors
Goldstein, Larry B.*	Medicine/Neurology	Stroke
Greene, Ronald C.	Biochemistry	Biochemical Interactions
Greenfield, Jr., Joseph C.*	Medicine/Cardiology	Cardiovascular Physiology
Hamilton, John D.*	Medicine/Infectious Diseases	HIV Infection
Lyles, Kenneth W.*	Medicine/Geriatrics	Metabolic Bone Disease
Madison, Roger D.*	Surgery/Neurosurgery	Neural Regeneration
Matchar, David B.*	Medicine/General Medicine	Health Policy
McNamara, James O.	Medicine/Neurology	Neurobiology
Morey, Miriam C.*	Medicine/Geriatrics	Rehabilitation
Morris, Kenneth G.*	Medicine/Cardiology	Cardiac Imaging
Piantadosi, Claude A.*	Medicine/Pulmonary	Pathophysiology of Hyperbaria
Postlethwait, Raymond W.	Surgery	Esophageal Pathophysiology
Pratt, Philip C.	Pathology and Laboratory Medicine	Pulmonary Structure
Pisetsky, David S.*	Medicine/Rheumatology	Autoimmunity
Quarfordt, Steven H.	Medicine/Gastroenterology	Lipid Metabolism
Seigler, Hilliard F.*	Surgery	Tumor Immunology
Simel, David L.*	Medicine/General Medicine	Quantification of Physical Examination
Sommer, Joachim R.	Pathology and Laboratory Medicine	Cardiac Structure and Function
Swartzwelder, H. Scott*	Mental Health	Neurobiology

Table II *continued*
Long-Term Investigators

Name	Department/Division	Research Interests
Turner, Dennis A.*	Surgery/Neurosurgery	Nervous System Aging
Weinberg, J. Brice*	Medicine/Hematology and Oncology	Monocyte and Macrophage Function
Weiner, Richard D.*	Mental Health	Electroconvulsive Therapy
Wilson, Kenneth E.*	Medicine/Infectious Diseases	Bacterial Identification
Wilson, Wilkie A.*	Medicine/Neurology	Neurobiology
Wilson, William P.	Mental Health	Electroencephalography
Young, Stephen L.*	Medicine/Pulmonary	Pulmonary Physiology
Zung, William W.K.	Mental Health	Depression

Thirty-three scientists are listed who have directed a research program at the DVA for a minimum of 20 years.

The asterisk indicates that the investigator was active at the DVA at the end of 2005.

Centers

In describing the research activities, the individual investigators have been grouped by their departmental affiliations. Many of these investigators also have participated in a number of research Centers. The membership of these Centers ranges from being localized to the DVA or DUMC through national and/or international affiliations. They have provided an additional avenue for targeting specific research endeavors. It is beyond the scope of this presentation to describe separately each of these Centers. However, they have been an integral part of the research effort.

Because of the size and complexity, two DVA Centers deserve a detailed description of the history and activities: Health Service Research and Development (HSR&D) and the Geriatrics Research Education and Clinical Center (GRECC).

HSR&D

One of the highlights of the research program of the DVA has been the rapid growth of the HSR&D Program[8]. In the autumn of 1981, Ramon Velez, M.D., M.P.H., Chief of Health Services Research Affiliation of Durham, N.C., applied for and received initial funding for a Health Services Research & Development (HSR&D) Field Program. The opportunity arose because leadership in the national HSR&D Service desired a more geographically dispersed system, one per VA region, and these would form the nexus of the new HSR&D. Each Field Program was expected to accomplish at least four objectives: 1) to conduct relevant, high-quality health services research; 2) to stimulate health services research and to provide technical assistance in its development; 3) to provide support and consultation to area managers and providers; and 4) to inform and educate VA managers and providers about HSR&D, its use and methods. Additional responsibilities included: 1) to serve as a VA system-wide resource in a selected priority area(s), and 2) to perform or assist with one or more such special functions as VA system-wide training, collaborative research, merit review, and evaluation and dissemination of research findings. Collaborative relationships with local institutions and research organizations were encouraged. The DVA Field Program established formal ties with Duke University Medical School and the University of North Carolina (UNC) School of Public Health.

During the grant application process in January 1982, B.F. Brown (Fred), DVA director, emphasized Durham's "unusual strength and potential" for one of the new HSR&D Field Programs. Durham was already a Health Services Research (HSR) Center and had a long track record of successfully competing for research funding and attracting highly competent investigators. Mr. Brown anticipated that Durham's unique position within the VA system would assure its success.

A goal, cited in the grant application, was the desire "to broaden our efforts at educating VA clinicians and health administrators in the uses and limitations of health services research, thereby helping to make patient management and resources allocation decisions in a more effective and efficient way. We hope to accomplish this by both developing appropriate didactic sessions and by actively involving staff in identifying problem areas suitable for HSR."

Also, there was an active interest, support and commitment of key clinical and administrative staff. Fred Brown saw HSR&D as a high priority for the hospital and expressed a strong need for the type of input HSR could provide, especially in the areas of district planning and the regionalization of patient referral patterns. Ramon Velez, then HSR&D Affiliation Director, had training in health services research and clinical epidemiology and had been active in the initial efforts to establish an HSR&D program. Kathryn Magruder-Habib, a Ph.D. in epidemiology from UNC and the new HSR&D associate director, was familiar with institutional resources and faculty at the UNC School of Public Health and would provide groundwork for a meaningful and constructive relationship with that University. Harvey J. Cohen, M.D. (Chief, Medicine Service, DVA) had been the Director of the Geriatric Fellowship Program, and was Director of the Division of Geriatrics and Associate Director of the Aging Center at DUMC. Shirley A. Beresford, Ph.D., an epidemiologist and biostatistician, was scheduled to join the staff in March 1982. John R. Feussner, M.D., M.H.S. (Chief, Ambulatory Care, DVA) had already successfully carried out several HSR projects. Edgar Cockrell, M.P.H. in health administration, had been chosen as the administrative officer for the program.

Both DUMC and UNC showed interest as well. Congruent with the HSR&D mandate, the Center for the Study of Aging and Human Development, the Department of Health Administration, the Department of Community and Family Medicine, the Center for the Study of Health and Clinical Policy, and the Department of Medicine at DUMC pledged support, coordination and collaboration in research and training. Similar support was tendered by the UNC School of Public Health, the Health Services Center, the School of Pharmacy, the School of Dentistry, and the School of Social Work.

When the Veterans Administration's Health Services Research & Development Program began to fund the new Field Programs in the spring of 1982, the DVA was among the first four Centers chosen. DUMC was the affiliated medical institution. Known as the Mid-Atlantic Health Services Research and Development Field Program, Durham was designated as Region 2 and encompassed 28 VA medical centers from New Jersey to North Carolina.

The Durham Field Program was to maintain a network of research and educational affiliations that included the Mid-Atlantic Field Office, the DVA, the Geriatrics Research Education and Clinical Center (GRECC), and various departments and research units at DUMC and UNC. It was designated as a system-wide resource in ambulatory care, disease prevention, and technology assessment, as well as a Ph.D. training site in health services research. The first budget was $123,300 for the 1982 fiscal year.

The Program's first year of operation acquired a staff of approximately 18. The core staff included Director Ramon Velez and John R. Feussner as M.D. investigators and Kathryn Magruder-

Habib, Shirley A. Beresford, and James A. Neff as Ph.D. Health
Science Officers and Edgar Cockrell as Health Science Officer and
administrator. There was an additional group of 12 research project and support staff and an additional five Ph.D. students.

Not everyone knew exactly what to do with this new Center. One
of the early requests for assistance from the Regional VA Office was
for assistance in better elucidating the most cost efficient method
for cleaning laundry across all VA sites. Should some laundry be
done at each facility, or should cleaning be centralized? Early leaders in HSR&D conducted a significant amount of education as to
the science, utility, and appropriateness of topics. The sophistication of the science of health service research grew both locally and
nationally.

By 1988, the Field Program's total budget had grown by more
than 1400% to $1,773,088 and the Program staff had grown as well
in both M.D. and Ph.D. researchers. Since 1984, Dr. Feussner was
the Field Program Director in the DVA Ambulatory Care Service.
Physician areas of training and expertise were in clinical epidemiology, biostatistics, decision analysis, technology assessment, and
meta-analysis, with specific clinical research interests in general-
ist/specialist differences in clinical practice, geriatric health and
physical fitness, outpatient disease screening (specifically in alcoholism, depression, and cancer), hypertension measurement and
follow-up, quality assurance, and the use of outpatient resources.
Physicians also maintained DUMC faculty appointments in the
Department of Medicine, Division of Internal Medicine. Increas-
ingly, the emphasis of the Program focused on the delivery of primary care to Veterans. Work done by these researchers would become the cornerstone for the future changes in the delivery of
health care at the DVA that occurred in the mid-1990s.

During this period, the number of Ph.D. researchers had grown
as well. Areas of expertise were in biostatistics, epidemiology, medical sociology, and health economics with research interests in the
areas of assessment of common and/or chronic disease, prevention and early disease detection, as well as access to ambulatory
care, the coordination of that care, alternatives to VA care, and
quality assurance. The Ph.D. staff were given appointments at the

DUMC Department of Community and Family Medicine, Division of Biometry.

The Program's research focus now was in three broad, yet interrelated areas: ambulatory care, disease prevention, and technology assessment.

In ambulatory care, the focus was on access to care, resource utilization, medical records systems as clinical and research tools, quality assurance, and chronic disease epidemiology with an emphasis on hypertension, diabetes, alcoholism, depression and psychosocial issues, and cerebrovascular disease.

The disease prevention focus encompassed primary and secondary prevention. One project was a nation-wide survey of priority research areas for disease prevention in VA Ambulatory Care programs. Also, there was research in introducing exercise and fitness programs for the elderly; early detection of hypertension, cancer, depression, alcoholism, and cerebrovascular disease, as well as spinal cord injury morbidity studies.

Technology assessment research focused on carotid artery disease and blood pressure measuring devices, monitoring mechanisms in diabetes mellitus, and measurement of hematologic variables. Research also evaluated the physician's bedside performance as a "diagnostic tool."

Durham also developed an M.D. and Ph.D. fellowship program which proved to be the major source for new faculty in future years. The M.D. fellowship program resulted from the establishment of a Division of General Internal Medicine in 1976 by James B. Wyngaarden, M.D., then Chairman of the Department of Medicine at DUMC. The program recruited M.D. fellows who were board eligible or certified, preferably in Internal Medicine, who acquired clinical training, and who expressed a commitment to careers in academic medicine. Preference was given to candidates with training in clinical epidemiology, biostatistics, or decision analysis and who had participated in research activities as evidenced by presentation of their work at national meetings, or by published articles or abstracts. The first of these M.D. fellows began in 1982.

The Center's Field Program for Ph.D. trainees became a source of strength and satisfaction. By 1988, the Program had 13 students, both post- and pre-doctoral status, all with a research emphasis on ambulatory care or disease prevention. They were chosen for their specific interests that were compatible with the Program's research goals. An HSR&D Field Program report in 1988 stated, "Most of our success in the doctoral training area has been with the School of Public Health at UNC." By 1990, 15 Ph.D. candidates had been sponsored by the VA Office of Academic Affairs (OAA) and DVA's HSR&D doctoral training program. The total budget for that year was $1,829,669.

Both M.D. and Ph.D. faculty in the Durham Field Program worked together to create the first Clinical Research Training Program at DUMC. There was a clear need for formal didactic training in clinical and health services research for the growing number of faculty and trainees. In most institutions, this didactic training occurred in their School of Public Health, but DUMC did not have such a school. DUMC, under the leadership of William E. Wilkinson, Ph.D. and Dr. Feussner, created the new training program within the School of Medicine in 1986. The degree conferred to successful students was a Master of Health Sciences. Early funding for this program was obtained from the A. W. Mellon Foundation. The courses and education were tailored to the needs of clinician researchers and the majority of the faculty who taught in this new Master's program were researchers in the Durham Field Program. By the end of 2005, and now under the leadership of Eugene Z. Oddone, M.D., M.H.S., this program has granted degrees to over 500 clinician researchers.

The Center continued to grow and pursue a diverse research agenda in the access, delivery, quality and outcomes of primary care. The Center owed a significant amount of its early success to a strategic link with health care delivery at the DVA. All physician investigators practiced medicine at the DVA and projects arose directly from their practice. The Center's Director, Dr. Feussner, was the first recipient of the Mark Wolcott Award for Clinical Excellence presented by the Department of Veterans Affairs. The Wolcott Award was established to recognize outstanding Veterans Health Administration health care practitioners who made contributions of national significance in the enhancement of health care. Though he was recognized for a number of contributions to VA health care, he was specifically recognized for "his desire for personal excellence in providing health care for his own panel of patients" and his record of ongoing, continuous achievements in the area of health services research. Also, in the late 1970s, "Dr. Feussner took the dramatic step at that time in creating a primary care model in the DVA" and therefore was primarily responsible for the DVA becoming a leader in primary care, research, and education. In 1994, the name for Durham's Health Service Research Field Program was changed to the Center for Health Services Research in Primary Care.

In 1996, the Center's Director, Dr. Feussner, left to become the Chief Research and Development Officer for the Department of Veterans Affairs, Veterans Health Administration. Dr. Feussner became the first national leader of VA research to set a wider agenda that emphasized the unique contribution of VA research to the health care and quality of lives of Veterans.

In 1997, the Center had over 30 full- and part-time staff comprised of M.D. and Ph.D. researchers, fellows, statisticians, and support staff. The 1997 Center's total budget was $3,677,829. Core researchers included David L. Simel, M.D., M.H.S., whose research focus was on clinical examination skills. He would become the major leader for a successful educational series in the Journal of American Medical Association termed the Rational Clinical Exam. Ronnie D. Horner, Ph.D., epidemiologist with expertise in neurologic diseases, was the Associate Director of the Center. He served as Acting Director during the search for a permanent director who would lead both the Durham Center and the Division of General Internal Medicine at DUMC. Dr. Horner's instrumental research led to a greater understanding of the epidemiology of stroke and stroke care in the VA. Also, he was principal investigator of an instrumental study that established a link between deployment to the Persian Gulf and later development of amyotropic lateral sclerosis (ALS). David B. Matchar, M.D., M.H.S., a general internist with expertise in decision sciences and health economics, also conducted his early research in the Center. His first VA study established a link between hyperglycemia and poor outcome for patients admitted with acute stroke. He would use these findings and his expertise to obtain one of the first large center grants in stroke prevention from the Agency for Clinical Health Policy and Research. Dr. Oddone, also a general internist, worked with Morris Weinberger, Ph.D. on one of the first VA Cooperative Studies designed to evaluate a health services intervention that tested whether access to an enhanced model of primary care could reduce hospital readmissions for Veterans discharged from the DVA Medicine Service. He also studied racial disparities in health care, publishing one of the first studies that established a disparity in utilization of carotid endarterectomy in the VA in 1993. Dawn T. Provenzale, M.D., M.P.H. a gastroenterologist, forged a successful career examining quality of care in colorectal cancer screening and treatment. Also, she formed a successful GI outcomes research group within the Center to which she has attracted several junior physicians to careers in health services. Hayden B. Bosworth, Ph.D., a research psychologist with expertise in gerontology, joined the Center in 1998. He developed expertise in interventions designed to improve patient adherence to regimens designed to control chronic disease, and he has successfully tested these interventions through both VA and NIH funded studies. He also served as lead author of the first text book written by Center investigators: *Patient Treatment Adherence: Concepts, Interventions, and Measurement.* Lawrence Erlbaum Associates, Mahwah, NJ 2006.

In 1997, Dr. Oddone took over as Director after having just completed an HSR&D Career Development Award. He charted a broad research agenda in primary care research in order to address diverse facets of primary care issues and the impact on Veterans. Research focused on health care delivery, outcomes of care, health care for women Veterans, medical ethics and patient preferences, generalists-specialists differences in the provision of health care, addictive substance research, and special problems in spinal cord dysfunction.

HSR&D investigators from Durham also attracted national attention for their research efforts. In the autumn of 2001, James A. Tulsky, M.D. was chosen for the prestigious Presidential Early Career Award for Scientists and Engineers (PECASE) for his work and research in physician-patient communication and the care of dying patients. This annual award is the highest honor bestowed by the

United States government on science and engineer researchers beginning their independent careers. The reviewers highlighted that Dr. Tulsky's research appeared in high-quality journals, that he testified before a Senate Special Committee on Aging, that he was the Associate Directorship of the DUMC Institute on Care at the End of Life, and he had a growing reputation as an expert in medical ethics and improving the care of dying patients.

In the winter of 2003, Dr. Weinberger received the highest award given to honor a VA health services researcher: the annual Under Secretary's Award for Outstanding Achievement in Health Services Research. The award was established in 1998 in recognition of the importance of the Department of Veterans Affairs health service research program and its vital link to the health care of Veterans and the public. Dr. Weinberger was the first non-HSR&D Field Director to receive this award. Dr. Feussner, the initiator of the Under Secretary's Award, said that "Dr. Weinberger stands above his peers with regards to his research productivity, his value as a health services researcher to the Department, his value to the research leadership within the VA as a policy advisor, and the leadership he brings to the health services and epidemiology research effort at the DVA. He embodies the character, innovation, persistence and productivity represented by the recognition inherent in this award." Dr. Oddone also received the Under Secretary's Award for Outstanding Achievement in Health Services Research. His seminal work in racial disparities linked with his studies on access to care were cited during the ceremony as having great national importance in helping the VA better understand new models of care.

At the end of 2005, the Center had over 140 full time faculty and staff. The M.D. and Ph.D. investigators account for over $9 million dollars in annual VA research funding, and an additional $6 million in non VA research funding. The Center has grown in sophistication as a research organization, consolidating expertise in information technology, electronic capture of information, national expertise in database management, and interventional research. The core area of emphasis remains access and delivery of primary care and the Center's greatest success is designing and testing interventions that improve access and quality of care for Veterans.

GRECC

Just after the launch of the HSR&D Program in 1981, Harvey J. Cohen, M.D., the ACOS for Education, DVA, coordinated a proposal to VA Central Office which requested funding for a Geriatric Research, Education and Clinical Center (GRECC) to be located at the DVA[9]. GRECCs are Congressionally-mandated "Centers of Excellence" designed for the advancement and integration of research, education and clinical achievements in geriatrics and gerontology for the VA health care system. The DVA GRECC was formally activated in March 1984 with Dr. Cohen as Director and a total salary budget of $238,000. The GRECC mission was to improve and expand the capability of the VA on a local, district, and regional basis to meet the medical, psychiatric, and social needs of the increasing number of aging Veterans and to foster an increase in the quality of geriatric care through research and training of health care personnel.

The reputation of the affiliated institution, DUMC, in the area of aging was already well established due to the presence of the first and longest continuously funded Center for the Study of Aging and Human Development in the country and the newly formed Division of Geriatric Medicine, both also under the direction of Dr. Cohen. These programs assured the new DVA GRECC of substantial support, visibility, and quality from the outset. Over time, the DVA GRECC significantly expanded into 8500 square feet of dedicated office and laboratory space. It has attracted outstanding professionals with national reputations in the field of aging to conduct basic, clinical, and health services research for the ultimate benefit of the aging Veteran. In 2005, and after two decades of research activity, the DVA GRECC remains under the direction of Dr. Cohen along with three associate directors and a multidisciplinary staff represented by medicine, nursing, social work, pharmacy, and dentistry. GRECC salaries currently total approximately 1.5 million dollars; GRECC investigators' research awards were approximately 22 million dollars.

In the area of *basic biomedical research*, GRECC investigators focus on the relationships between cancer and aging, cardiovascular disease and aging, and immunology and aging. GRECC laboratory programs have focused on enzymology of the aging immune system and transcriptional regulation of protein kinase. Dr. Cohen's research helped to elucidate lymphocyte membrane and cellular responses to stimuli in the elderly. The groundbreaking studies of Lina M. Obeid, M.D. helped to establish the role of ceramide in cell senescence. More recently, studies of Gregory A. Taylor, Ph.D. have described the regulation of host resistance to intracellular pathogens.

GRECC *applied clinical research* targets patterns of cancer in the elderly, comprehensive assessment of the gero-oncology patient, exercise for cardiovascular fitness and mobility, and reduction in impairments from osteoporosis and Paget's disease. Notable GRECC clinical studies include: The Development of a New Measure of Balance ("Functional Reach") by Stephanie A. Studenski, M.D., M.P.H., Miriam C. Morey, Ph.D. and others; Osteoporosis and Disability in Life Care Community Women by Kenneth W. Lyles, M.D. (both funded by the Claude D. Pepper Older Americans Independence Center for which Dr. Cohen is the Principal Investigator); Depression in Medically-Ill Veterans by Harold G. Koenig, M.D., M.H.S.; Disability in Nursing Home Residents with Dementia by Eleanor S. McConnell, Ph.D.; The Varicella Vaccine Trial for the Prevention of Herpes Zoster and its Complications led by Kenneth E. Schmader, M.D.; The Treatment of Impairments and Bone Remodeling in Aging Patients with Paget's Disease, and Hip Fractures in Elderly Men by Dr. Lyles and Cathleen S. Colon-Emeric, M.D.

GRECC *health services research*, with a general focus on health promotion and disease prevention, involves studies on the evaluation of geriatric care models, drug utilization in the elderly, and investigations of informal caregivers of elderly Veterans with chronic illness, including their economic burden and quality of life. Illustrative examples of GRECC Health Services investigations have included: The Impact of a Geriatric Consultation Team in an Acute Care Hospital (Drs. Cohen, Studenski, and others); The Impact of the Gerofit Program on Health and Fitness (Dr. Morey); Trajectories of Health and Service Use among Aging Veterans (Elizabeth C. Clipp, Ph.D.); and Medication Use And Health Outcomes In The Elderly (Joseph T. Hanlon, Pharm.D., M.S. and Dr. Schmader). National Health Services trials include: The National

Longitudinal Caregiver Study led by Dr. Clipp; The National Geriatric Evaluation and Management (GEM) Trial led by Dr. Cohen; and the VA Stroke Rehabilitation Services and Patient Outcomes Study led by Helen M. Hoenig, M.D., M.P.H.

Clinical and Health Services research in Rehabilitation began programmatically via the Geriatrics Program when Dr. Studenski became Chief of Rehabilitation in 1986. She developed a research program focused on falls and dysmobility, working jointly with co-investigators in the Duke Department of Physical Therapy. Research by Dr. Studenski and colleagues led to the first Duke Claude Pepper Center. At least three of the physical therapists with whom she collaborated earned a doctorate degree and remain active in rehabilitation research. Pamela W. Duncan, Ph.D. is internationally renowned for her research in stroke rehabilitation. When Dr. Studenski left in 1992, Dr. Hoenig, also a geriatrician, was recruited as Chief of Rehabilitation Medicine. Dr. Hoenig has facilitated a highly collaborative rehabilitation outcomes research program. Results of work by herself and other rehabilitation researchers at the DVA led, in part, to the second DUMC Claude Pepper Center, establishment of the VA Rehabilitation Outcomes Research Center in Gainesville, Florida, and the NIDRR Rehabilitation Engineering Research Center on Wheeled Mobility in Everyday Life in Atlanta, Georgia.

Currently, active funded rehabilitation research at the DVA includes: studies of exercise for osteoarthritis of the knee (Kelli L.D. Allen, Ph.D.); changes in gait in elders with various diseases (James T. Cavanaugh, Ph.D. and Dr. Morey); functional recovery after acute stroke (Larry B. Goldstein, M.D.); novel methods for evaluating dysphagia (Carol S. Hammond, Ph.D.); telerehabilitation for persons with mobility disability, measures of rehabilitation quality of care, and the impact of mobility aids on functional outcomes (Dr. Hoenig); exercise counseling to improve function in older patients (Dr. Morey); changes in joint and cartilage with arthritis (J. Brice Weinberg, M.D.), and executive function deficits after stroke (Sandra D. Zinn, Ph.D.). Rehabilitation researchers at the DVA now span the spectrum from physician and post-doctorate fellows to junior faculty and senior faculty.

Facilities

One of the continuing hallmarks of the DVA Research Program has been the plague of inadequate research facilities[10,11]. When the hospital opened, only one area, Building 10 (2500 sq. ft.), was dedicated for research (Figure 1). There was immediate clamor from the professional staff to develop additional research space. The initial Hospital Director, Horace B. Cupp, M.D., made available approximately 2000 sq. ft. of reasonable wet laboratory space on the second floor of the hospital which was quickly occupied— but fell far short of the need. In fact, throughout the five decade period a significant number of the Merit Review funded DVA investigators have carried out their research endeavors at DUMC.

An Animal Care Facility, Building 14, became functional in the 1950s, and provided space for the care and maintenance of a variety of animal species. However, procedure and operative space was not adequate to meet the increasing needs. A variety of areas within the hospital had to be utilized as operative and procedure areas for large animal research. In addition, a number of projects requiring the use of rodents were carried out with these animals housed within the hospital proper. Obviously, these arrangements were not ideal, but were functional. By 1960, the burgeoning research program was in dire need of additional space.

Clinical research on human subjects was carried out in various clinical laboratories. As examples, the Cardiac Catheterization Laboratory was utilized to study ventricular mechanics and the Pulmonary Laboratory housed a sophisticated study of capillary blood flow.

As the research program grew, research space was obtained by converting space within a number of small buildings which had been built for other uses. The first of these, Building 5, had been constructed as sleeping quarters for the nursing staff but was made available to the Research Service. It became the initial site of the Cooperative Lipid Laboratory developed by E. Harvey Estes, Jr., M.D.

The amount of space available for research through the early 1960s is difficult to determine. As noted, much of the research was carried out within the hospital in rooms frequently used for other endeavors as well as research.

In 1967, the only dedicated space designed for research was opened—the E-wing of the hospital (Figure 2). This wing contains 17,000 sq. ft. of usable research space. This building was devoted to wet laboratories and large animal studies. The opening of the E-wing fostered considerable consolidation and allowed many of the investigators who had been scattered throughout the hospital to be housed in one location. However, as might be anticipated with the continued growth of the research program, by the time the E-wing opened, it was clearly inadequate to meet the needs. Thus, a continual effort was made to acquire additional research space.

Two buildings originally constructed for living facilities, Buildings 2 and 4, were renovated in 1970 and 1981, respectively. When refitted, they contained approximately 4,000 sq. ft. of reasonable research space. Building 4, occupied by the Infectious Diseases scientists, was used for the AIDS Center and in 1993 was augmented by the construction of a P3 biocontainment unit.

In the mid 1980s, the DVA consolidated the Laundry Service which moved to a central location. This building was acquired by the Research Service, renovated and currently is in use by Nephrology and Immunology.

The construction of the Extended Care Facility, which was opened in 1989, did away with Building 5 but added approximately 3,000 sq. ft. of research space which supports the GRECC Program.

Building 16, constructed in the 1970s as an Education Center and office building, was acquired by the Research Service and houses a considerable portion of HSR&D and Neurobiology Research.

Additional hospital space was obtained when the clinical laboratories were consolidated. This includes office space for the Research Administrative Staff as well as approximately 2,000 sq. ft. of laboratory space.

Although funding had been previously approved to renovate and expand the Animal Care Facility (Building 14), the project was stalled. Through the dedicated efforts of John D. Shelburne, M.D., Ph.D., ACOS for Research and Development, and Conrad Richter, D.V.M., the DVA veterinarian, this outstanding animal facility was completed in 1998 (Figure 3). This facility consisted of 20,000 sq. ft. of space. In addition to the animal care components, there is approximately 5,000 sq. ft. of research space utilized by a number of investigators.

Currently, the total usable laboratory research space available for investigators on the DVA campus is approximately 39,487 sq. ft. In addition, the HSR&D staff utilize approximately 10,295 sq. ft. of space for their endeavors. In addition to the E-wing and the hospital space, the remaining research laboratories currently are housed in six separate buildings.

At the present time, two Merit Review funded investigators have their research program housed at DUMC.

What should be obvious is that every conceivable square feet of available space for research within the DVA campus has been utilized. The research facilities are not ideal and suffer considerably from the isolation of the various laboratories in a number of different buildings and in some cases, substandard construction.

The DVA Research Service has been informed that construction of a modern biomedical research building has been approved in the VA Central Office. Construction should begin in 2008. The current plan is to locate the facility next to the Vivarium and near the main hospital building (to the right in Figure 3). The completed building will consist of five floors, each containing 10,000 gross sq. ft. One floor will be finished initially. The additional four floors will be added as funds become available. Although the final completion is well into the future, this building will be beneficial in allowing some consolidation of the current research enterprise as well as providing a very significant increase in new laboratory space.

Figure 2

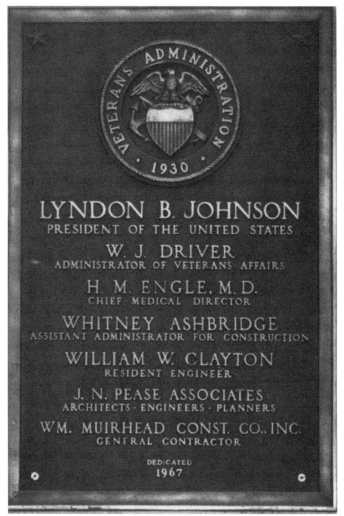

This bronze plaque dedicated the formal opening in 1967 of the
Research Building designated as the E Wing.

Figure 3

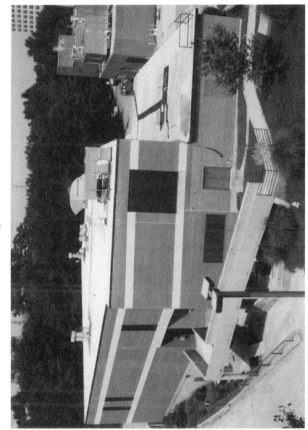

This modern animal facility was completed in 1998.
It contains both the original structure (Bldg. 14) and a new addition.

Funding

One of the key aspects of any successful research program is to secure appropriate funding. From the inception of the program, the DVA investigators relied primarily on three sources of funding: the VA, the National Institutes of Health, and industry. Without a significant amount of money from each of these sources, the program could not have achieved its impressive growth. During the initial years of the program, VA monies were by and large obtained directly through personal contacts in Central Office. The initiation of the Merit Review Program in 1967 and the establishment of a peer review system enabled the VA investigators to compete directly for funds.

Unfortunately, the precise amount of yearly funding during the initial period is unavailable. In Table III, the yearly expenditures are listed—beginning in 1982 and for each five years thereafter. (The last row gives the 2005 figures.) Data provided include: research support from the VA, Medical Research and HSR&D, as well as other non VA sources such as the NIH and industry. Also, the total funding is listed. It is clear that the DVA investigators have been extraordinarily successful in obtaining research funding. The total yearly research funding at the DVA consistently has been within the top tier of the VA Research Programs.

In 1988, the DVA Research Service made use of the public law authorizing the Department of Veterans Affairs to establish private nonprofit organizations to provide a flexible support mechanism for research. Thus, the Institute for Medical Research (IMR) at the DVA was created. The IMR is a state chartered, 501 (c) (3) nonprofit entity which administers funding from industry, foundations and governmental agencies. The primary mission of the IMR is to support the DVA Research Program through numerous avenues including: purchasing equipment, updating laboratory space, fostering a small grants initiative, and providing training opportunities for personnel. The overall function and direction of the IMR is overseen by a Board of Directors. Membership on this board is mandated through congressional guidelines and consists of four statutory board members (Director, Chief of Staff, ACOS for Research and ACOS for Education from the DVA) along with two community representatives. In addition, there are usually four at-large members. Currently, approximately $2,500,000 in assets are deposited in the IMR.

In 1998, the IMR began to fund a small grants program. The purpose of these grants is to provide "seed" money to support pilot projects which enable the DVA scientists to obtain additional funding from the VA Merit Review Program as well as from the NIH, industry and foundation grants. Since its inception, three to seven grants ranging from $15,000 to $17,000 have been funded each year. To date, 35 grants have been funded—bringing the total expenditure to $539,000.

Investigators at the DVA have been extensively involved in a number of projects within the Cooperative Studies Program. The level of funding from this source has increased markedly during the past decade and for 2005 is $1,582,494.

A very important mechanism in the growth of the research program has been the judicious use of the Career Development Program. In fact, the DVA Clinical Service has been heavily dependent upon this mechanism to support not only research, but the clinical enterprise. An interesting paradox arose from the very successful acquisition of these awards in that the number of staff funded physicians, especially in the medical subspecialties, was never adequate to meet the clinical needs. Thus, the Career Development Program has been an essential mechanism for carrying out both research and to support patient care.

The Career Development Program contained four different levels: Associate Investigator, Research Associate, Clinical Investigator and Medical Investigator.[12] Associate Investigator Awards were obtained by 15 physicians. Six of these later were appointed as Research Associates. Thirty-four additional physicians were awarded a Research Associate position bringing the total to 40. Twenty-seven individuals were awarded Clinical Investigator positions. Of these, six had been Research Associates. Four physicians were appointed as Medical Investigators. The HSR&D Program has a separate Career Development Program and 11 physicians have received one of these awards.

The original Career Development Award Program was phased out in 2000 and a new program initiated which is targeted at junior level investigators. The new Career Development Award (CDA) Program contains only two levels (Level 1 and Level 2). Currently, at the DVA, there are three investigators at the CDA Level 2.

Several years ago, the DVA instituted a competitive program to fund the salaries of Ph.D. investigators working in the VA Research System. Currently, there are five Research Career Scientists at the DVA funded through this mechanism. In addition, HSR&D supports a Career Development Award Program for Ph.D. scientists at several different levels of accomplishment. Five individuals at the DVA receive support from this program.

Table III
Research Funds

	Medical Research	HSR&D	Non VA	Total
1982	2,086,700	123,300	816,000	3,026,000
1987	3,894,700	425,900	2,281,000	6,601,500
1992	4,966,100	1,204,300	6,995,600	13,166,000
1997	5,337,300	1,360,400	4,277,900	10,975,500
2002	8,544,400	5,236,400	8,169,700	21,950,500
2005	6,883,300	9,263,600	8,134,400	24,281,300

The approximate value of research funds at the DVA are listed in dollars (not adjusted for inflation).[13] Funds derived from VA sources are listed in Columns 1 and 2. Column 3 lists the funds of all non-VA sources. In Column 4, the total research funds are given. Of note is the dramatic increase in research funding for HSR&D.

Administration

For a program of similar size, the administrative structure of the Research Service at the DVA Hospital was unusual: for the first 25 years there was no Associate Chief of Staff (ACOS) for Research and Development. As noted, the Administrative Officer for Research and Development throughout this period was Burley H. McCraw who reported directly to the Chief of Staff. Burley was extraordinarily effective in organizing the various components of the research program as well as dealing effectively with the VA Central Office to obtain significant research support. Burley was instrumental in developing the strategy which ultimately resulted in the building of the E-wing—the only space constructed specifically for research on the DVA campus. Truly, Burley, by any yardstick, is the "unsung hero" of the Research Program at the DVA. In 1982, Mr. Jim Duncan became the Administrative Officer for Research and Development and continued in Burley's footsteps to enhance the administrative structure of the program. In 1992, Mr. Larry Freeman was appointed and continued effective leadership until August 2003. In the spring of 2004, Mr. Bradley Olson took over the helm. In 1978, the first ACOS for Research and Development, Gerald L. Logue. M.D., was appointed—followed by John D. Shelburne, M.D., Ph.D. in 1981 and Stephen L. Young, M.D. in 1992. In 1999, the current ACOS for Research and Development, J. Brice Weinberg, M.D. was appointed.

Throughout the existence of the research program, the administrative functions have been outstanding. In fact, many of the investigators have volunteered laudatory comments regarding their support. Committee structure consists of the following four subcommittees as components of the Research and Development Committee: 1) Institutional Animal Care and Use Committee 2) Institutional Review Board 3) Subcommittee for Research Safety

(includes Radiation Safety) 4) Research Space Committee. These
Committees have functioned efficiently and effectively in the various administrative duties.

Future

The Research Program at the DVA continues to be an extremely vibrant and growing concern in spite of the difficulty experienced in obtaining adequate research funding during the past decade. The investigators have been extraordinarily productive and show every indication of continuing this path in the future. As always, the quality of the research will be driven by the expertise and dedication of the people involved. The leaders of DUMC continue to make a major effort to provide a cadre of excellent scientists to carry out research at the DVA.

One major problem remains: a pressing need for consolidation and updating research space. The future direction of the Research Program will be negatively influenced unless a viable solution to this problem is forthcoming. Hopefully, the proposed 50,000 gross sq. ft. research building will help alleviate this problem. Unfortunately, the final construction will not be completed for a number of years. At least, for the foreseeable future, the very significant problem with inadequate research space will continue.

Securing a workable, timely solution to the space problem, coupled with the attitude and expertise of the current scientists at the DVA, leaves little question that the future will continue to be, as in the past, outstanding.

Sources

1. Personal interviews with a number of research scientists and administrative leaders: Thomas M. Coffman, Harvey J. Cohen, E. Harvey Estes, Jr., Ronald C. Greene, John D. Hamilton, Rodger A. Liddle, Christine E. Marx, Jonathan B. Mark, Claude A. Piantadosi, Hilliard F. Seigler, Joachim R. Sommer, Richard D. Weiner, Wilkie A. Wilson, William P. Wilson, Christopher W. Woods, William E. Yarger;
   ACOS' for Research and Development: Stephen L. Young, J. Brice Weinberg and Timothy Hammond;
   Chiefs of Staff: Thomas F. Newcomb and John D. Shelburne;
   Administrative Officers for Research and Development: James Duncan, Larry Freeman and Bradley Olson.
2. *Durham Morning Herald,* Sunday April 19, 1953, VA Hospital Section. Devoted to describing the construction, staffing and dedication ceremonies.
3. Report of a site visit which determined the need for Part II funding, May 15, 1968, chaired by Harold C. Wiggers, Ph.D.
4. A listing of the Department of Medicine Faculty assigned to the DVA were obtained by Sandra G. Mangum from the Departmental records.
5. A bibliography of each investigator was obtained from the National Library of Medicine and National Institutes of Health via PubMed (www.pubmed.gov).
6. Other biographical information was obtained via www.google.com.
7. Greenfield, Joseph C. Jr. *Duke Cardiology Fellows Training Program-Origin to the Present*, Carolina Academic Press, Durham, N.C., 2004.

8. History of the Durham Health Services Research and Development Program (HSR&D) (written for this overview by: Eugene Z. Oddone, M.D., M.H.S. (Chief, General Medicine, DUMC); Edgar Cockrell, M.P.H., Chief Financial Officer, HSR&D; and Steve Wade, Librarian, HSR&D).

9. History of Geriatric Research Education and Clinical Center (GRECC) (written for this overview by Elizabeth C. Clipp, Ph.D. and Harvey J. Cohen, M.D.)

10. Synopsis of the Research and Development Service, Durham VA Medical Center (written by Stephen L. Young, M.D. 1992).

11. Research News—Department of Veterans Affairs, March 1994.

12. Marguerite T. Hays, M.D. researched the available data in Central Office and provided a comprehensive list of the Career Development Awardees.

13. The current administrative staff of the Research Service, HSR&D, and the Institute for Medical Research provided vital data on space utilization as well as finances.